Too Many Tears

Too Many Tears

Susanne Moss

Preface by Pierre Berton

McClelland and Stewart Limited

Dedicated to John Howard Griffin,
author of *Black Like Me,* with all my love.

0-7710-6566-3

McClelland and Stewart Limited
The Canadian Publishers
25 Hollinger Road, Toronto

PRINTED AND BOUND IN CANADA

Contents

Acknowledgements

My deepest gratitude goes to Pierre Berton, who, despite an excruciatingly heavy schedule, found time to sympathize with my aims and inspired me to complete my story; to Mr. Adrian C. Adamson, Chairman of the Social Sciences and Humanities Department at Humber College of Applied Arts and Technology, and Dr. Wallace Northover, Chairman of the Faculty Council at Atkinson College, York University – two men who believed in me, bore with me, and helped me through the many problems; to Joseph Tatarnic, long time friend and confidant and always available for help; to Richard Ketchum, Father Clark, Fr. Thomas McKillop, Mrs. Patti Nagy, Mrs. Mary Powers, and the staff of the Metropolitan Toronto Central Library.

Many of the names
of persons and places
in this book have been changed.

Preface

Susanne Moss is a brave, lonely and bitter woman. She is bitter because she is locked inside a prison from which she can never escape – the cage of her own body; it is this which makes her both lonely and brave. She is lonely because she has few friends, because communication with the outside world is difficult; because locomotion is ungainly and it is not easy for her to be close to anyone. She is brave because she refuses to accept passively the strictures of her condition: she insists on operating at a level which would seem to be beyond her apparent capabilities. This often leads to frustration and to more bitterness but, exhausting though this struggle must be, it is her only hope.

Many people, on meeting Susanne, think that she is drunk. Her words are slurred and distorted. Because she cannot control her muscles, her face goes out of kilter. She walks awkwardly and with considerable effort. Policemen have sometimes tried to run her in, believing her to be intoxicated. This, understandably, drives her into a fury.

Others, on meeting Susanne, think that she is mentally retarded. They talk to her as they would to a child and this infuriates her still further. Or, worse still, they refer to her in the third person – conversing over her head to a companion as if she did not exist. All handicapped people face this unthinking excommunication. Blind men and cripples have told me that when they enter a restaurant with their spouses, the waiter does not talk to them. "What will he have?" they ask the wife, as if blindness or lameness was somehow to be equated with imbecility.

Susanne Moss, as this book shows, is an intelligent and literate woman, with an IQ higher than the average. Her attempts to get an education, against the will of her parents, friends and even some of her teachers, must have been Herculean. All of her life she has struggled to control her infirmity often in the face of well-meaning resistance. One of the problems she faces is that many people cannot believe she is able to do some of the things she does. How can this woman, who can scarcely get a cup of coffee to her lips, make her own clothes and type a book-length manuscript?

Frankly, I do not know how she does it. She lives alone in a high-rise apartment and she has no help. She cooks all her meals. She has cooked meals for me and very good they were, too. She makes excellent shortbread. In short, she lives as normal a life as she can manage. And yet, anyone acquainted with cerebral palsy must understand how exhausting simple household chores must be for her. Simply to type a page of manuscript on her special machine with the indented keys, takes four or five times as much energy as it would for you or me. Yet she manages it because she must. Susanne Moss has no intention of becoming a vegetable.

Off she goes doggedly, out the door, down the elevator, along the street and into the bus – often enough the subject of inquisitive stares – to deliver her lectures at Humber college, shop in the supermarket, or to spend time with friends.

These excursions often bring their own trials. Constant exposure to public gaze has made Susanne hyper-sensitive. With the best intentions in the world, people often say or do the wrong thing – and sometimes they can be downright cruel. Sympathy is the last thing Susanne wants. She rejects it grimly. When other women call her "dear" or "you poor thing" (as other women often do) she is capable of real rage. She is not something to be petted or patted or wept over. More than anything else she wants to be treated as a human being and as an equal, to be scolded for her imperfections as much as praised for her strengths.

This book, which has been a catharsis for her, was a long time in the making. It began as a result of a letter she wrote to me, typed by herself and signed with her wavering hand. The letter resulted in a remarkable television appearance – the first time, I believe, that a victim of cerebral palsy had ever been interviewed on the medium. That half hour program, forthright and moving, produced a wide and positive response. As a result, I urged Susanne to develop some of the things she said on television into a longer work.

Over a period of many months she produced a typed manuscript. After that, with some help from her publisher, she rewrote it entirely. Susanne, of course, is not a professional. In her manuscript she made all the errors that beginning writers are prone to make. The manuscript was too long. There were the usual digressions that got in the way of the real story. There were things left unsaid and other things that needed to be clarified. This is where Rick Davey, a talented young writer, entered the picture. He took Susanne's story, trimmed it to size and with her active help and encouragement moulded it into its present shape. To a very large extent the words are still hers; the story, of course, always has been. But it reveals a great deal about Susanne Moss to know that it was at her insistence that Rick Davey's contribution to this book be acknowledged here. Susanne's affliction may cause her to totter a little from time to time, but she is, as this story reveals, a woman who insists on standing firmly on her own two feet.

PIERRE BERTON

Introduction

The clock in the corner grocery read four-fifteen. I stopped and leaned against the steamy window. I was tired and cold. Winter whistled along Bloor Street, it blew a candy wrapper past my feet. The chilling March wind attacked the aging buildings. In front of me two dogs skulked against the lashing gusts, their eyes squinting and their jowls blowing back from growling teeth. People walked with their heads down, hands clenching scarfed necks.

Larry and Jill would be wondering what had happened to me. I pulled the collar of my new coat closer around me – I had been so proud of it an hour earlier, now it was only shelter. I would have cried but there were no more tears for that kind of thing. I tugged my hat more snugly over my ears. It was just a few blocks to a warm apartment and friends. I started again: I followed the two dogs.

Larry and Jill had just moved from a second-floor walk-up in the annex. I used to have trouble getting up to that flat, negotiating the narrow winding staircase with its slippery and worn steps. I was relieved that I wouldn't have to go through that.

I pulled open the glass door of their new apartment building. I struggled with the wind and finally managed. The elevators waited for me, whisked me to their floor.

Jill and Larry were waiting at the door.

Susanne, what a lovely coat!

I couldn't respond to her friendly greeting.

What's wrong? You look dreadful.

I just wanted to sit. I would sit and take off my cold boots. I'd feel warmth, then I'd tell them.

The tears were closer. Humiliation is always the worst. The rest I can fight. At last, I told them what had happened.

I can see her still, standing above me in the cold and crowded bus, her fat gloved hand jerking to the bus' bumping while it seized the metal support. Above me, her nose red from the cold winds, her powdered brow, her expensive fur hat. Eyes, so accusing, damning my physical disability. And her penetrating voice:

You poor, sick thing.

The ignorant questions, the emphatic statements.

Are you always in pain? How did you manage to get to church today? You're so helpless.

Someone had intervened. It was a loud male voice.

Shut up, lady! Leave the girl alone.

I couldn't even thank him. I got off the bus at the next stop and walked the rest of the way.

Larry was angry.

Who was this woman, Susanne? Have you ever seen her before?

Yes. She always sits in the front row at church. I've seen her quite often. But she's never even said hello to me before.

We sat in the homey living room, the three of us in a circle of furniture. What could be said? Perhaps there were once words. Maybe there still would be if this had been just an isolated incident; ignorance and stupidity can be forgiven to a certain point.

I am thirty-seven years old today. I have lived all these years with spastic cerebral palsy. I have seen and done, heard and thought like anyone. And I have laughed and cried, but I have cried too much. Yet I have never suffered physical pain from my disorder.

My handicap is descriptively simple: my muscles contract when I try to make any complicated movement. It is not as bad as it once was – not since my discovery of Valium, a drug that relaxes the muscles – but still I am restricted and retarded in my physical ability.

The years have forced me to make allowances, to adjudge

situations and face the restrictions that they force. All my actions are slower and appear more unstable than they really are for I must be careful, less so since a new drug, but still. . . . Still, cups must have a handle large enough to allow my thumb a secure hold; glasses must be small enough for a firm grip, and thick enough so that my tight grasp will not shatter the glass and bloody my hand. Always I take a half cup and a half glass for I would spill a full quantity.

I used to have to grip my fork like a heavy hammer and hold my meat with my left hand to steady it against my uncertain attack. Now I use less of the hand; if the meat is soft I can use a knife but I hack rather than cut. My manners are not the refined movements that etiquette teaches. They never will be.

Not even the new drug can completely overcome the spasm that is my condition. My hands bunch themselves into small, rigid, almost robot-like devices, the muscles stand blue and hard preventing me from grasping the small zipper handles and tiny buttons on the backs of dresses. My hair style is dictated by the fact that I cannot manipulate rollers.

Always there has been a struggle within me. I know that I must be careful, slowly cautious in all my movements, in all my actions, but there also is a driving force that insists I be self-sufficient, that I manage on my own. Yet every task takes so much longer than it does for the physically whole person. When I dust or wash the windows, I must hold the can in one hand and push the spray nozzle with the other; I have to hurry to catch the liquid before it dries, useless to my task. I put on my makeup, I bake and cook, I do all the house cleaning in my apartment . . . slowly. Very few things are automatic; movements must be weighed for security against bodily harm. The oven is left to cool before I remove my dinner; most of my household containers – cosmetics, cleaners, food – must be unbreakable.

I have never been reluctant to talk about these physical problems. I have been forced to accept my handicap. That part of my story seems much less important than another part. I have sometimes thought that I would manage well enough if it were not for these other problems – if life were not a social experience. It has always been people that have made things difficult. They apply a pressure with their hostile gazes or their looks of pity. They heighten the inherent tension of my handicapped body, drive me involuntarily to spastic responses.

My cerebral injury affects my speech; it is somewhat difficult to comprehend and few people make an attempt to understand. Store clerks assume that because I have an impediment I am incapable of making purchasing decisions. People insist on anticipating my needs rather than listening to my own requests. These are the maddening types of frustrations. This is where the hurt is.

Writing this book was a gigantic physical undertaking for me. I had to struggle with smudgy sheets of carbon, with the spasm in my body that made finding the right key at the typewriter a long and frustrating task. But even more difficult was the necessity to re-live the emotional hurts I have experienced. Sitting alone at my typewriter was much like the existence I have known – physical problems mean very little beside the ugliness I have encountered moving my spastic body within society.

Now the book is written. The experiences have been re-lived, the keys have been hit, and the carbon has become garbage. My story is told. But it is my story only in that the specifics are mine. I share a common suffering with many handicapped people. This is their story too. We cry from frustration. Tears are our bond and this is for all of us.

Susanne Moss
Toronto, 1973

Part I

Part I

The first seven years of my life seem sketchy and unrealistic to me today. There were so many things that I didn't understand – and there was always the constant fear. I was always protected, always addressed with a mocking tone of voice. I was either "you poor sick thing" or the dreadful family curse. I don't remember much kindness; there were the endless visits to doctors in a hope of finding a cure or at least some reason for my physical defects.

There are things that I can remember; others I cannot. There are so many "what ifs" attached to my early childhood days. What if Tom and Rose Moss had been more educated, what if . . . but . . .

I was born in 1935, the middle of the Depression. The arrival of a child was not a joyous occasion for my parents; it was a difficult time for a young European couple with little education. Tom had his dollar-a-day job, Rose had the church. They spoke no English.

I have seen my friends in this expectant state – the mothers proud of the life they hold in their wombs, the fathers who have a boastful twinkle in their eyes. But Rose Moss had no pride. Even later I can remember her shielding my eyes when we passed an expectant mother on the street. She would explain that the woman had sinned.

Birth, in her terms, was the result of sin; its process was one of mystery. I have asked my mother many times about this lack of knowledge. Her explanation was always the same, always incredible.

She could not go to school because she was needed on the farm. But she did go to catechism for four years, twice a week, so that she could make her first communion. The priest told her that she must never talk about babies being born. That was a sin. On the farm she saw how chickens were born; that was the extent of her knowledge.

From friends my parents learned that when the pain started, Rose would have to go to the hospital. I have heard her explain to others, curious as to the circumstances of the sick child's birth and ignorant of the processes administered in the large red-bricked hospital:

When the attendants took me from Tom's side and . . . and they started to get me ready, I was petrified. They took all my clothes off and started to wash me and shave me. I started to yell, "Tom – Tom – help me." But they continued cleaning me as though for a feast. I really believed that they were going to butcher me. When they got me clean enough, they put a backless gown on me. I nearly died of shame. Then they put me on a bed and rolled me into a big room. There were white sheets hanging from the walls. I continued yelling, not so much from pain as from fear. They gave me a needle, then another, a doctor came, uncovered me and gave orders to take me into the operating room.

White dressed figures stood all around, their faces covered. I tried to run; they tied me to the table, then gave me gas. I woke up and they were still washing off the blood. I should never have seen the blood.

And so I entered the world with the blood which should never have been seen – the offspring of an hysterical, ignorant woman, obsessed with fear and shame. Somehow an oxygen blockage had damaged cells in the muscular cortex of the brain. In cerebral palsy cases, this area is injured before, during, or after childbirth.

I can never know the exact cause of my handicap, but I do know that my mother underwent severe mental stress from the time she entered the hospital. There were medical reasons.

But for Tom and Rose Moss their child's disorder seemed only God's wrath:

Oh Tom, we should have saved our money so that we could be

married in the church. She is our curse.

I can remember being taken to parks to play in the thick grass or the small green sandboxes. My mother would meet her friends and sit under a tree on the chipped wooden benches. I was always close to her, always just a few steps away.

I existed, even then, as a puzzle to curious, ignorant minds. How many times did I hear Mother explain the details of birth? How many times did I hear her friends ask about her poor sick child? And then after the details:

Oh, Mrs. Moss, it's such a pity. You will have to live with the shame for the rest of your life.

Yet I never *felt* sick. I noticed, of course, that I could not handle things the way others did. It was true that I had trouble playing with my rubber balls or my soft rag dolls. I found it so frustrating to try to fill my pail with sand with my little toy shovel. But after many attempts I could do it. And I found that the more I worked and practised doing any one specific thing the better I could do it. I could even walk at three. It was an unstable walk; I tottered from side to side, but I walked – towards the other children. I just wanted to play with everything as they did, to join that excited laughter that was always so far away.

I was always lonely on those trips to the park. There were other little girls and boys. When Mother and I arrived, I saw them laughing in the sandbox or running in the grass, but when I approached them, their mothers would decide it was time to go home. First they would ask my mother how I felt, then they would take their children away. I was left alone with my soft toys and my bewilderment. And with the imagined horrors that my Uncle Edward kept suggesting.

All my memories of my father's third cousin are accompanied by an irrational terror. I remember his ruddy, angular face, the thick brown hair, the lips that never smiled, the eyes that always accused. His presence was the dominant memory of my earliest years.

Edward had arrived in Canada from Europe to escape his country's draft about five years before my parents emmigrated. His ambition had taken him far in the new world. He had mastered

English within a year of his arrival, and by the time I became aware of an Uncle Edward he was a very successful real estate agent.

There were reasons for my parents to appreciate and depend on the interest Edward showed towards them. His success brought friends and acquaintances of similar background, while his knowledge helped my parents to understand the goings on in a country that communicated in an unknown language. He was always the fourth member of the party that consulted with the English-speaking doctors.

But to Edward this constant searching for a diagnosis was a useless exercise. His solution was both straightforward and unceasing – there was no question but that I should be placed in an institution and forgotten about. I was a curse to the family.

And most of the doctors had no better answers. Some concurred with Edward – the most sensible thing would be to have me committed to an institution. Cerebral palsy, at that time, was an unknown disease. The symptoms were all too often identified with mental retardation.

I was unaware of what the doctors said, since they never talked in front of me, but I could tell a great deal from my parents' words afterwards, from the pain on their faces. Some nights I would lie awake in my bed and hear them discuss the doctors' reports with visitors. There was always Edward's constant message:

See, I told you she's worthless. Now the doctors have proved that she's possessed by the devil. See, they told you point blank to send the creature where such ones are kept. How much longer must this family suffer from the shame you have brought it? Send her away at once. Only then can you be saved. Do you hear me?

And there were the other visitors.

Remember the Doblins? They had a little sick boy like your Susanne. Last winter, one night when it was below zero they put a piece of wood in his mouth and tied him to a tree in the yard. He froze to death before it was dawn. No one saw what they did. You know Dr. Jacksi will sign any death certificate for twenty dollars. Stop torturing yourselves and do the same thing. If you are afraid that the undertaker might think that you are responsible, do what the Patriskies did with their crazy girl. They bound her and covered her with snow in the wood shed; it looked like she was playing too long in the snow. Everyone took their word for it. Just remember to cry as long and as hard as you can; that's what everyone does when they don't want to be suspected of doing away with their rotten children.

Fortunately, my mother would not hear of any of these remedies to cure the family curse. As far as she was concerned my disability was the fault of the doctor who delivered me. The effect of these attempts to take her daughter away was almost as injurious to her mental health as it was to mine. Finally, even the sight of Edward would cause her to become hysterical.

In a further attempt to learn more about my handicap and in a futile plan to escape the domination of Edward, the family moved to Toronto in 1939. Perhaps in the city there would be more doctors who spoke our language. Surely in Toronto there would be some answers.

No.

The usual response was that indeed I was a sick girl. No, there was nothing that could be done. Just take good care of her.

So began the phase of overprotection. There was nothing that I was allowed to do on my own. I was either carried everywhere or held in a firm grasp when I tried to walk. I was dressed, fed, bathed, and fussed over. My muscles were allowed exercise only in the dark that surrounded my bed at night.

It might have been different without Uncle Edward, without his ignorant determination. It might have been, but it wasn't.

Even when there were times of hope, times when I heard grown-ups speak things that were not confusing but seemed to make wonderful sense to my curious young mind, he would turn hope to hopelessness, happiness to gloom.

One of the doctors that my parents took me to was Dr. Allen Brown, one of the pioneers in the medical diagnosis and treatment of cerebral palsy in Canada. I visited him just before my fifth birthday. I can still remember his smile while he examined me, his firm hands that never hurt, his long white jacket that smelled like soap. He waited till I was ready before he told my parents, through the interpretation of Edward, what he thought. I heard his words, the first ones that had made sense to me. Of course, he was right. Yes, yes, the longer I played at something, the easier it was. Tell them again, Dr. Brown. I must be given the right kind of exercise, lots of it and good food. I would improve; I would overcome my handicap completely.

I don't know what became of Dr. Brown's diagnosis. It could be that Uncle Edward did not translate it properly. It could be that my parents had given up long before this, finally convinced that my case was hopeless or perhaps it had gone too far for them. Maybe to them this was just another in the endless futile series of foreign words and waiting rooms.

I remember my fifth birthday and the arrival of my mother's brother, Michael, and his wife, Helen. They brought me gifts, dresses of bright colours with lace at the collar and sleeves, and matching stockings. They brought me toys, a new doll with blond hair and a red dress, and a picture book of funny animals I had never seen before. They brought me smiles and laughter. I don't remember them asking me how I felt once. (Although they did tell my parents that Mother's family was upset about my condition.)

And there was a crisp white dress, with frills and a pink ribbon in the front. This was to be the dress I would wear for my baptism. Helen and Michael had come to be my godparents.

There was a birthday cake for dessert that night but I don't remember eating any of it. Uncle Edward arrived during dinner. He started yelling the moment he was introduced to Uncle Michael.

What's this crazy idea I hear about you coming all the way here to have this thing baptized?

He called them as crazy as me. He threatened to have me committed to Orillia without my parents' permission – he said that he could do it just by swearing to some form and paying a doctor to do the same thing.

I never wore the dress with the pink ribbon and there was no baptism. Michael and Helen left later that week; they said it would be better to allow the situation to calm down without them. But nothing really calmed; there were only my tears when they left.

But this time Uncle Edward had overplayed his role. I didn't see him again for many years. Such threats and the stories of torture were too much for my mother; she would leave her Tom, she would take me and go if Edward was ever allowed in her house again.

There was no longer fear and anxiety with me in my bed at night. They were replaced with loneliness and a strange neglect. Not the neglect that comes from being ignored. No; it was the neglect of being taken for granted. I was excluded from all normal activity.

My sixth year was a year of good fortune for Tom and Rose Moss. My father won a sweepstake; dollars and dollars of good times. But I was never invited nor expected to share the excitement that swept my parents. The happiness was for everyone else.

What would have happened if the timing of things had been just a little bit different? What if my father had won the three-thousand-dollar sweepstake a year or two earlier? Would some of the money have been used to treat my disorder?

I watched them, saw the excitement a sudden windfall brings to a couple who have always struggled. I saw the apparent generosity that such good fortune created. Or was it generosity? Perhaps they saw only salvation, the opportunity to make up for the shame and humiliation that they brought upon their family and friends. The three thousand dollars was used to buy back the esteem they had lost when they produced me.

There were parties two or three times a week with fancy cakes and laughter. There were gifts for all the friends who had not deserted them and gifts for those who had. Uncle Edward and his family received a great deal of the good fortune. It was little thanks for all he had done. Even my mother agreed with this, although he was asked not to come to the flat to express his gratitude.

I lay awake in my bedroom. No one talked about me anymore. Everything was clear now. There were no more gruesome tales of children being done away with, no one spoke of insane asylums. They talked about the old country, they discussed the war, they spoke about their children. They laughed and sang; they danced on the waxed hardwood floor, their feet pounding to the clapping of their sweaty hands. I lay awake; sleep was impossible. I exercised my spastic muscles. It was all I had, that and my thoughts.

To add to the deliverance that Tom and Rose felt, Michael and Helen had a baby daughter. Lilian was a normal child, she was pretty, she was the greatest gift that the family could receive. Here was a little girl who would, who could be all that I could not. The Mosses went on another spending spree. There must be gifts sent to her – as many as possible; nothing would be spared. God had forgiven them. It was now so clear and uncomplicated.

I wondered why I couldn't even have a new doll.

I was left out of so much that year. So much, but they couldn't keep me out of everything.

My father was offered a job as a training superintendent in his company. There would be a new factory established in Woodstone. They asked him to move there and assist in the general training of new employees in the plant. It would mean a new home in a new town.

It was April when we moved – on a cold dreary day, more winter than spring, the air filled with a cold rain and a heavy wind. The house stood, unpainted on the wide lot, small in the dirty snow and wet leaves from the previous fall and winter. The gray, chipped front door looked hardly welcoming but this was the Moss' first house. Inside, the yellow linoleum floors curled to the dirty, peeling walls.

But our new home came to life with the approaching spring. I watched as my parents whitewashed the walls and laid bright new covering on the floors. The grass in the backyard grew green and thick with the warm rains and the sun. Soon flowers appeared in the garden, the green sprouting buds unfolded before my excited eyes.

It was my job to water the garden; it was my first responsibility. These were my flowers, this was my garden and it was beautiful.

It drew the children of the neighbourhood and brought me friends – friends who my mother chased away.

They were English children. My mother had a mistrust of the English, as she called everyone who spoke the language. It was decided that a fence would be put around my yard. I protested.

But Ma, they are nice girls. I like playing with them.

Shut up. You're sick and don't know nothing. They're no good for you. You must only play with our children. There's lots of them around the corner. Why don't you ask them to play with you?

But their mothers would never allow these children to come to my backyard.

The fence was built. Seven feet tall, my cage surrounded me and my flowers. Sometimes if I thought my mother was busy I would open the gate and let my friends in but she was never that busy; she would come running out of the house screaming words that these children could not understand. But they understood her meaning well enough; soon I was completely alone. I had my lovely garden but it could never be shared.

In the fall of that same year, my father received an invitation from Helen and Michael; they wanted him and me to come and visit them at their farm in northern Pennsylvania. They realized that because of the new responsibility of the house my mother would have to stay home, but couldn't Tom and Susanne come down for a long weekend?

Mother was reluctant to stay home, especially with the knowledge that we would see her niece while she wouldn't. However, Michael's concern about the house certainly made sense. She would stay home and father made arrangements to take two days off work. We left on the train Wednesday evening.

The first thing that Friday morning we were on our way to an institution in Rochester where Michael and Helen had arranged an appointment. They had learned that crippled children were actually cured there. Even my father felt some of the hope and enthusiasm that my aunt and uncle expressed.

It must have been a new building. I remember the bricks were white like new snow and the front door was all clean and glass, like looking in a mirror. I was examined by several doctors. After the final one finished inspecting my scrubbed body, a nurse helped me dress and showed me into a large office. My father and my aunt and uncle were sitting on a couch. The last doctor, the spokesman for the group, sat behind his desk. He smiled at me when the nurse brought me in; he had been waiting for me.

His voice was friendly but professional. All the doctors agreed that all I needed was the right exercise and a correct diet. My handicap was entirely physical, due to an injury to a part of the brain. I don't remember if he named the affliction but he did suggest that the best results would be achieved if I were placed in the institution for the next five years. He was fairly confident that my handicap would be completely overcome by the time I was twenty if these steps were taken.

He presented my father with a chance; it was my chance for a normal life. It wouldn't be tomorrow, or the next day; it was a long way away. I turned to watch my father's reaction and saw the indecision in his eyes. He spoke English very well by now. He understood what the doctor had said.

At that moment I knew that he wanted me to be well. But there was little hope for any chance. Uncle Edward's words filled the room; they choked my father. He knew that my mother would never allow me to be placed in an institution. He thanked the doctor; he said that he would certainly discuss it with his wife. We left the institution to return to my uncle's farm.

We spent the next three days at the mink farm. No one ever discussed the visit to the doctors while I was around. It soon left my mind; I was too absorbed by everything around me. I would watch the minks in their crowded cages or I would help Michael feed the chickens. I was fascinated with the pigs and one day I even rode the old sway-backed horse. In the evenings I helped my aunt with Lilian. She had big brown eyes and fair hair; she would kick her arms and legs and smile and laugh when I leaned over her crib.

We went home to mother on Sunday. We went home to tell her what the doctors had said. I don't remember my precise thoughts, certainly Uncle Edward's words had not escaped my memory, but surely that kind doctor would not torture little girls. I wanted to be better, to have friends, to be loved and not endured.

But there was never really any question about her reaction. My father knew it and I guess I did too.

No. No. Never. I would never be taken away from her. I was part of her flesh. This was the last time that any such nonsense would ever be discussed. The doctors were all crazy. No one was going to torture Susanne.

That was the end of the search. Uncle Edward had not achieved his objective. I would never be abandoned to the imagined tortures of one possessed by the devil. But by the time I was seven there was little hope that I would escape my own private hell.

Woodstone did not provide any relief from the boredom and loneliness that all the other places had offered. There can never be anything else when a mind, growing and struggling to emerge, is presented with only the most simple occupations. My mother would drag me around Woodstone, through the shady treed streets and the small downtown shopping section. Often when she would stop to talk, I would wander a few feet from her side, to gaze at everything around me. Oh, if only I could join those children who were running across the street. But I never could; there was always my mother's hand grabbing me as hard as she could. Wouldn't that hand ever let go?

There was the sandbox in the summer but the ridiculous simplicity of such activities no longer amused me. In the winter there was nothing but the walks in those bulky clothes that seemed to choke me at every step, shielding me from all the world, not just the cold of the season.

At home there were still the simple toys, the soft rag dolls and rubber blocks, so used, so worn out, so juvenile. Why wouldn't my mother let me help her do some of the cooking? I used to watch her – the eggs, the flour, all those things in the bottles, into a bowl, into the oven and then out again. I was fascinated, but

I could never help; I could only watch.

There were only a few times of emotional warmth. It never came from my parents, nor from any human source. But I can remember going to people's homes and watching the family cat. While my parents sat and talked to their hosts, the cat would slowly come creeping towards me. Something live, warm, cuddling, purring in contentment to my slow petting – only cats have been this.

When we first moved to Woodstone; Woodstone and our first house, the large backyard, there was a kitten for Susanne. I named her an unoriginal Pussy. She was a friend, confident, release. She was Pussy, black and white clean fur in my lap, at the bottom of my bed. She was the first emotional involvement I can remember.

And then there was the radio, my educator, my companion – that makeshift model, which, my parents informed me, some engineering student had thrown together just before I was born. It never worked very well, especially after we moved to Woodstone, the crackling static was louder than its strongest signal; even the large Toronto transmitters had trouble sending their programs to our home. But somehow they managed. My father would come in from his day at work, and after what seemed too long a wait, the receiver would faintly and then more strongly awake to his decisive turn of power. And then the voice of Jim Hunter on CFRB: "And now the news."

My parents would sit in awe of the great voice, in appreciation for its coming into their lives. I would sit and listen with them. This was ritual, this was the way things happened in the Moss household. Dinner would wait until the end of the news.

But one evening my father attempted to decrease the annoying static of the machine; I watched as the radio became a mangled heap of tubes and wires which was then placed into a fixed pattern on the dinner table. But then father was stuck and his frustration grew as he realized his inability to arrange the same pile back into what was once a radio.

My mother and I laughed at his futile attempts. After many curses, he finally realized that there was no solution but to purchase another radio. Yes, we would meet him at the Simpson's mail order shop on his way home from work. Yes, we would order a new radio, a good one, with lots of bands. There was a program on from the States in the afternoon that was in our language; it would have to be strong enough to pick that up; perhaps, it would be good enough to get something from the old country. It certainly would have to bring Jim Hunter into the kitchen.

The radio was ordered. We waited through quiet evenings, through early dinners, me and Pussy, my mother and father. And then it came – in a cardboard box that my father said was very heavy. We waited as he unwrapped the protective casing. His hands disappeared into the box and then emerged with that beautiful oak case, the black front, the dials, and the numbers. It was placed on the table, the antenna was attached, the power turned on. Jim Hunter's voice crashed through our house with the awesome power of the German infantry that he was describing. Pussy jumped and ran away in fright. My father turned down the volume. Everyone smiled.

Today the media has become a rather blasé form of entertainment in our society. Every child is born and reared to the television. But to me, in the early 1940's, it was the beginning of an exciting new phase of my life.

It is difficult to explain the position that the radio held in my early life. It was friend and challenger, educator and entertainer; it taught me English so that I was able to understand the language completely and without strain. It didn't matter as much that my parents treated me like an imbecilic vegetable, the radio was the same to me as it was to everybody. It played the music, it transmitted the serials, it informed about the war; it never told me that I was sick, that I should be sheltered from the world.

I hummed with Frankie Sinatra on the *Saturday Night Hit Parade,* laughed with Arthur Godfrey. I lived in the backstage with Larry in *Backstage Wife,* preferring the evening shows like *The Alderich Family* and *Our Miss Brooks* to the more syrupy afternoon shows – *One Man's Family* or *Portia Faces Life.* I dissected the news with Walter Winchell, questioned some of his opinions in my eager and private way.

It became important to me that I should not miss any of my favourite programs. This forced me to learn how to tell the time and read a calendar. At each station break, when the announcer would give the correct time, I would look at the kitchen clock to determine the setting of the hands for this particular time; in the beginning I made mistakes, but my mother helped a little, and soon I was able to determine what numbers looked like and how to tell time as well.

The calendar presented the same problem – the solution was based on the same pattern. Our kitchen wall was covered with merchants' calendars, the beautiful settings, snow on mountains or clear streams through lush green valleys. My mother explained the charting of the calendar, how the numbers were arranged under the days in groups of seven. Soon I knew what the names of the days and months looked like and I could distinguish all the numbers up to thirty-one.

After such education came the more exciting gifts of the radio. I would listen to the stories, hear the place names of cities, their chief characteristics and places of interest described in such a way that forced my young mind past the edge of a stilted reality to the excitement of imagination. I would lie awake in my bed and see the monstrous proportions of the Empire State Building, its upper stories reaching past the clouds; or I would imagine myself in the backstage of a famous theatre, with the costumes, the stars, the rush and excitement that I just knew had to exist in such a setting. It never concerned me that I might be incorrect, that my imagination might be running wild with ridiculous fantasies. No, this was all too new and exciting to bring it back to the drab little house in Woodstone.

And certainly the radio brought me much more than just the exciting world of the stars; there was a war raging and despoiling Europe. There was lots of news about this. I would hear the English commentators decrying the autocracy of the German nations, and praising the brave young men who were dying to save mankind from the tyranny Hitler threatened to all men. But it was a confusing war to a little girl. I would listen with my parents to an afternoon program they would occasionally pick up in their language on the short-wave band. I would hear these commentators exclaiming that the English under Churchill were committed to the destruction of Europe.

Perhaps this confusion was good too. Today I find it difficult to find any fault with the radio of my youth. Yes, I certainly disliked some of the programs while others bored me because of their simplicity, but all of them made me feel that I was part of the world. For seven years I had lived with useless toys, with fear, and without the impetus necessary for the development of my mind. The radio gave me hope.

I deserted my few toys; Pussy grew bored with me and found a new friend in the old Quebec stove, while I sat beside that wondrous wooden box staring transfixed at its light.

Fear and hostility gradually disappeared. There were still incidents when I was painfully reminded of my handicap; there was still an underlying uneasiness in my home; but in the main, through the next thirteen years I began to expect more of life.

My cat and then the radio provided the first hints of this change. After affection and then involvement, my mind demanded more opportunities. I wanted to be like those distant children. I soon found that the only way I could expect anything other than pity and aversion was to speak up – I had to let the world know that I existed and that I was not "sick." I wanted things – love, friendship, stimulation, responsibilities. I knew I was capable, my only problem was convincing my parents of this fact.

My chance came when my mother determined that the Mosses should embark on a program to make our house more comfortable. Mother took a job at one of the many new factories that were changing Woodstone into a modern suburban community. Shifts were arranged so that I would never be left alone, but still this new family schedule released me from my mother's bondage. I was given responsibilities; I washed the dishes, I fed my cat. The garden became more mine than ever. There was also more time alone with my father, who it seems, in remembering back, was less protective than my mother.

I remember being with him in the backyard one afternoon. He

was busy pouring cement for the new cellar walls and not in a position to run into the house to find out the time for himself. I guess it was just a mental lapse on his part, but he asked me what time it was. I embarked on the errand joyfully – imagine my father asking me what time it was – and returned to tell him with all the exactness that I could master, the precise time of the day, adding in a small show of pride that he had better hurry if he meant to be to work on time. He freed himself from the task and ran in to check for himself; I don't know whether he doubted me or whether he was just guarding himself from any letdown or show of surprise. I was right. But of course I was right; if I couldn't tell the time how could I have followed the radio programs so regularly and without missing one? He was overjoyed. He grabbed me and held me, asked me how I learned such a thing. Certainly it was no big deal for me to know that I was right, but this was the first time that anybody had congratulated me for anything in my entire life. My father was pleased, proud, and happy; I had made him feel that way!

Just before Christmas there was a similar occurrence with friends who came to exchange greetings of the season. I was sitting quietly in front of the radio listening to a program, quite resigned to being left out of the conversation as I had always been. One of the guests, a young woman, left the gathering and came over to join me. She asked if I listened to the radio often, what programs I liked, and other questions. When she learned of my interest and my genuine knowledge of the more popular programs and current events, she was delighted. We continued our conversation through the afternoon.

When Christmas Day arrived, this same lady sent me colouring books and cut-outs with my favourite radio stars in them. It was a different Christmas for me. There were still the silly and very juvenile toys, there were still the dresses, all far too big. But there was also these new presents; those voices that I had learned to know so well had faces and they were on my lap. There was a cut-out Ed Gardner of *Duffy's Tavern* and a drawing of Jack Benny with his squeaky violin. I was amused by the caricature of Bob Hope, the nose that was much too long, the exaggerated slope;

and I wondered how such a voice could come out of the skinny, sunken-cheeked Frank Sinatra. The Christmas candy that was a regular gift to me, the still-common question of how I felt – they didn't bother me that year. I worked with my new possessions; it was difficult, my spastic fingers had trouble guiding the crayons within the lines, my cut-out figures possessed lumps and hollows which the characters did not deserve, but in time, as with everything else, I was able to master the art of colouring and cut-outs; so much so that my mother took me downtown to choose new books when these were finished.

That summer the town began construction work on the gravel street that ran in front of our house. I watched with the rest of the children in the area. We watched as the men and machines transformed the grass ditches and bumpy roadway of Elm Street into a modern paved road; we shared all the creeping movements of the large machinery, the bawling of the foreman, the not so gentle rebuffs of the workers.

These children asked me why they hadn't seen me at school. School! This was a relatively new thing for me. For years I had watched children file past our windows with their brown paper bags and their books, but it was all quite mysterious to me. I told them so. They didn't understand, quite naturally, but they were certainly helpful in filling me in on the brutality of the institution. That summer I learned that recesses and lunch were by far the greatest thing about school, that arithmetic was torture, but art was okay, as far as anything at school could be okay. There were a few of the children who voiced quite an opposite view; they assured me that school was fun, that reading and spelling were just great and the teachers were very nice people. Generally they were overruled by the more boisterous of the group who were quite vehement in their opinion that the only thing that school did was prevent them from sleeping in the mornings, playing baseball in the summer and hockey in the winter.

But I was curious about this place. They told me that it was called Emerson Public and that it wasn't far away. One day I went for a walk of discovery. I found the school easily enough, it was quite an old building, brick red; there were big cages in the playground beside it, and rows and rows of bicycle racks. It seemed pretty empty and deserted. I decided to return at a later time.

My chance came in early October. I made the same journey, arrived at the same location, and found much to my bewilderment the same apparent lack of activity that I had encountered on my first visit. This surprised me. I sat down and wondered about this problem. Then the bell rang and the stampede started. I hurried out of the way of the running children, the boys dashing for those big cages in the field with their baseball gloves and mitts; the girls to their skipping ropes, or to a corner in groups for little conversations. I spied a woman, she must surely be a teacher, I concluded, and with a daring which surprised me as much as it must have her, I asked her if I could come to school.

She was quite at a loss, but after regaining some of the stern countenance that she projected when I first saw her, she asked me to stay where I was. She would get the principal. I wondered what this principal was like, but still I stayed where I was, and soon a tall, slim man approached me with a smile, which was lucky, because I think that at that time my courage was just running out.

So, I hear you want to come to school.

He held out his hand in greeting and introduced himself as Mr. Harris. I asked him if he was a principal. Indeed he was, he said, then asked me who I was.

Everything was straight in minutes. He assured me that he would come to my house the next day and talk to my parents about my coming to school.

I didn't tell my parents about this meeting with Mr. Harris. (When I had told my mother about my visit to the school in the summer she told me that they didn't teach sick kids and that I had better stop wasting my time by walking all that way.) I grew excited about his promised visit. I just hoped that my father would be home when he came, and that Mr. Harris would come.

He did. Mr. Harris asked my father why he hadn't contacted the Department of Education. My father could only answer that he didn't know about such matters and stated his belief that there was nothing that could be done for children who had any type of handicap. But my father was so wrong. Mr. Harris noted that there were some crippled twins who lived quite close to us who came to school and participated in classroom activities like any of the other children. He advised my father to contact a Mr. Dobbs, the supervisor of schools. We were assured that Mr. Dobbs would be able to make some arrangements for my education.

Father was busy until November, but as soon as he was able, he made the visit to the supervisor. The very next day Mr. Dobbs came to see me. I liked Mr. Dobbs, I liked the way he talked to me, the interest he showed in my colouring books and cut-outs. We talked about radio programs and my desire to go to school. I was nine years old at the time; it would be difficult to send me to kindergarten, but when I demonstrated my ability to tell the time, the date, and to count, he decided that a home teacher would be a better idea. This type of program, he told my parents, would enable me to start school in a later grade and not be too far behind children of my own age.

One could hardly have made a more unsuitable choice of an initiator into the process of education than the portly and authoritarian Mrs. Mills. From the first moment she walked into our house I didn't like her. I didn't like the haughty attitude she showed towards my mother. I found her approach toward the willing student like that of a trainer towards a dog. When I did well with my assignments she would pat me on the head and then turn to my mother, the owner of this beast, and congratulate her on my progress. When I had trouble with certain things, as I certainly did, she would accuse me of laziness, and then, as though in second thought, excuse herself for the outburst. I was handicapped; she wouldn't let me forget.

But I loved her too, not the person, certainly not her constant reference to my handicap or her perfunctory teaching, but the fact that she was, that she came twice a week for two hours and brought with her everything that had been so hidden. She brought me reading, Dick, Jane and Sally; and numbers, the magic of totals. It didn't matter that I winced everytime she addressed me with her mechanical "dear," or that she ignored me for the confused and unenthusiastic parent who was present. All that was important was that I was learning and that I enjoyed it, that my brain was being tested and was able.

Mrs. Mills continued her teaching through that year and then resumed her duties the following fall. I had advanced a great deal in that one year, achieving competence in elementary reading and arithmetic and showing an ability to understand history.

But in the early part of the new year, Mrs. Mills received word from the government that her son had been killed overseas. It was, most understandably, a major emotional shock for the lady. The routine and responsibility of her teaching duties were too much for her to bear, and on orders from her doctor she was relieved of her teaching.

Her replacement was tall, slim, pony-tailed Miss Frost. My parents disapproved. They disapproved the lack of severity in the replacement's demeanour, the stylish clothes, the happy countenance. They had come to expect a teacher to respond to them, to keep them informed of my progress. Miss Frost ignored them.

But I could hardly disapprove of Miss Frost. I remember her as both beautiful and dedicated to me, not to my parents, not even to the authorities. Her first action was to throw out the Board of Education's books, the books that Mrs. Mills had been using, and to replace them with material she thought would be more interesting and worthwhile. We read *Anne of Green Gables,* played games using arithmetic, discussed what we heard on the radio. Everything had more meaning; she was not only a teacher but a friend. Often she would stay over the two hours to listen to a radio program with me.

But Mrs. Mills returned the following year. She was no longer the same severe Mrs. Mills; all that had seemed perfunctory was now more zombie-like. She would often lapse into states of total disinterest that would both annoy and scare me. She would excuse herself and say that she had been thinking of her son; often she would spend the entire session talking about him. I didn't know what to do. I knew that my progress was being hurt. My desire was to be able to start school the following September. I worked harder on my own. I tried to bring Mrs. Mills out of her lethargic trances; I even begged her to have Mr. Dobbs come and examine my progress.

He finally came. He asked me questions, examined my workbooks, and interrogated Mrs. Mills. Finally his face broke into a smile.

Well, Susanne, you've made it.

I turned to look at my mother. Her smile was a mask of disbelief.

What do you mean she has made it? You mean that she can start school?

Yes, the fourth grade.

The fourth grade. I was going to the fourth grade. I will never forget the happiness of that moment. It was the first time I felt the complete goodness of happiness, the first time the world seemed a fine place.

I was excited about going to school, eager to continue this learning experience in a formal atmosphere; but I was anxious as well, and just a little bit scared. There was no doubt that I could cope with the scholastic part of the new environment. I had enough faith in my own ability, and there was the assurance of Mr. Dobbs that I was ready for such a step. But I was twelve years old, unused to the constant company of children, and certainly backward in any social niceties that, however simple and common, are nonetheless part of the everyday life of a school atmosphere.

The Department of Education had done all they could in preparing me for one part of this life, but they were unable to acclimatize me to the other.

There was nothing I could do but wait for opening day and hope that everything would go well. I wanted to be liked, to have friends, to share in the activities of the school as much as I was able. Only time would reveal if my hopes could be fulfilled.

Emerson Public was closed for renovation and expansion for the first part of my first year; I would have to begin at the oldest school in the city, farther away and outside of the boundaries of my discovered territory. Mother took me the first day. We walked the blocks and blocks with the other children, the other mothers with their much younger children.

Mother climbed the old tumbling steps with me to the massive wood door marked GIRLS, opened it and then left me to the dirty walls and the unfamiliar surroundings. I found my way to someone who could take me to my room and introduce me to my teacher. Once in the room, I was left waiting in a desk at the back. Perhaps, I thought, I would like to continue with Mrs. Mills for a little longer.

Then with the ringing of the bells everything changed. The room was instantly filled. There were "hi's" to me as the charging youngsters hurried to their seats and cajoled others so they could sit with someone else. Noise, activity – just like the radio had made me think it would be.

My first teacher was Miss Huck. When I had been introduced to her she had just waved me to the back of the room with an occupied hello. Now, her first words introduced me. It was simple and short; I will always appreciate that moment.

The girl at the back of the class is Susanne Moss. It happens to be her first day at school because she wasn't as strong as the rest of you and couldn't start school sooner.

I was part of the class. I was told about my responsibilities: not to be late, to bring a note if I was sick, to take care of my books and keep my desk neat.

I found the friends I wanted; the acceptance that I so longed for, the participation that I envisaged. There were times when it was difficult to be sure. I would hear the sly remarks when I tried to walk down the hall, and my physical characteristics caused problems that first year. I was tall and relatively heavy, with an almost fully developed bust, an oddity in my own class where most of the other children were at least two or three years younger than me. I was also a little disillusioned about the building where I spent my first months in school – it was not the most comfortable setting for a twelve-year-old beginner. The old school was filthy, the toilets didn't flush, the walls were cracked and pealing, and outside if you leaned against the school, bricks would quite literally fall at your feet.

But I let them fall unnoticed. Many things were overlooked. I viewed the world, my school, my teachers, the new friends through a happy haze. Just the fact that I was at school was enough, and when, in the new year, I started at the rebuilt Emerson Public, the filthy washrooms were lost, like so many things of times before, in the happiness of my being. The sly remarks did not last long; fortunately, they never became blatant ridicule. In time, I did not even mind my mother's grip during the walk to and from school. If I could have skipped, expressed my joy in a physical way, I would never have stopped. It was the beginning of a wonderful period of laughter and sharing and fulfilment.

God, but it was wonderful to live an almost normal life. I am told that everyone, or almost everyone, looks back on their school days as something very special and I am certainly not an exception. I don't mean that there were no problems, that suddenly my handicap disappeared, for it certainly did not. But those years seem to come together now and I can't remember the hurt and frustration that has always been with me. I had problems. Yes. And I cried. But then, doesn't everyone? . . .

I finished public school when I was sixteen. I progressed with or surpassed the children I had started with through the grades and the advancing degrees of difficulty. I had friends and responsibility.

There was never any question in my mind that I would continue to high school. I had earned that right and I looked forward to this continuing step with excitement and anticipation. I knew that it would be different. The size of the place filled me with awe, and I heard with everyone else that there was a real difference, that the teachers were more friendly and the students were given more independence. This excited me, but it also worried me, for I had been treated with a certain amount of consideration in public school and I hoped that this would continue without any hints of patronage.

It would be a good summer. There was the garden to take care of, and of course the new world that had been unfolding with my ability to read more and more complicated books. There was a certain warmth as well, the warmth from parents, who, although they did not really understand, knew that all their worst fears about their child were unfounded.

But suddenly I was briefly plunged back to that other time before school, before the radio and the dignity that I had gained in the years after. It is hard to remember the incident, it happened so swiftly, without warning. I was sitting in the garden, with my parents, enjoying the sun and the smell of summer flowers. I heard the gate open, the decisive slam of the visitor, I turned and there from thc past, from the nightmare of a youth that seemed so far away, stood Uncle Edward. He had not changed, the sneer was still painted on his narrow lips, his eyes had gained no warmth over the years, his speech was still as haughty.

He ignored me, directed his words to my parents. They had gone too far, it was bad enough to allow me to go to public school, but high school was something that only the very special could enjoy. The shame had been great enough. There would be no reprieve from God if I was allowed to continue my education.

I went into the house. The horror of the scene, his ranting, my mother's crying, my father's pleading was too much. I didn't want to be near him, he had hurt me enough already.

But please, Father, please don't listen to him.

I heard my father threaten to call the police if he didn't leave. I can only assume that this was enough for Edward; he left. He never returned or at least if he did I never knew about it.

In late August Mr. Dobbs phoned me. He told me that he had made arrangements for me to meet the principal of the high school. Dr. Kester came to visit the week before school started. Unannounced he stood at our front door, a large man with blond hair and a most charming smile. He congratulated me on my achievements in public school and then, with an unforeseen gravity and concern, asked me about my plans and hopes for the future. It was the first time anybody had asked me that simple question, one so common to most young people.

What do you want to be?

I was thrilled with his concern and with my first chance to offer my response. It was well thought out or so I thought. The product of all the hopes and fears and suffering of a handicapped sixteen-year-old.

I told him that I wanted to be a lawyer, that I thought this was the best way for me to work so that others would not be hurt as I had been. I wanted to make laws so that doctors wouldn't hurt people the way I had been hurt. (I have always thought it much to Dr. Kester's credit that he did not correct my naivité, but rather was fascinated and pleased that I had set my goals so high.)

He explained the major differences that I would find in high school. There would be nine periods and I would have to move from class to class. There would certainly be problems in this kind of system for me, especially in the crowded hallways. He suggested that for the first year I join a class of slow learners who did not move as much from class to class. The subjects would be the same, he assured me, but there would just be fewer of them.

The meeting ended. Dr. Kester took his leave and, with the same goodwill that I remember him by, assured me that his time was available and that if anything came up I was to go and see him.

My father accompanied me to school that first day, through the crowded halls, the rows of lockers. He seemed so out of place, more awed than I was. I was frightened that morning, frightened of the people and the cold remoteness of the place.

I was just as frightened in my home room. I didn't know any of the other students, and the teacher stood, cool, and authoritarian at the front of the room.

Class started. Miss Ball, the teacher, turned out to be anything but the reserved person she appeared, and these garrulous students became my friends and helpers. With Miss Ball's initiation, students volunteered to help me through the halls when a move was necessary. I was asked to join these girls in my class, and then others for lunch and spare periods.

I smiled most of the time.

There was just so much to like at Stephenson High. The atmosphere of the place led you to believe that you were growing up: things were much more informal and yet teachers seemed to respect their students. I couldn't get over being addressed as Miss Moss when a teacher asked my opinion on some point.

There was Mr. Dicks, the vice-principal, liked by all the students for his fairness and interest. There were the assemblies, where every week we would gather, the entire school, in the auditorium. There might be a student skit, or sometimes a political speaker who would favour us with an informative, if a bit too long-winded, speech on some facet of government.

The assemblies broadened me, and the social contact of high school forced me to a more intelligent outlook. It was almost impossible to hide in the ignorance of my home and the way I had been brought up. I can remember, for example always being told that dark-skinned persons were somehow inferior – there were inferences that even to come in contact with a Negro or an Oriental would lead to some kind of disease. But during my first year a Japanese boy was elected president and a Negro, treasurer of the student body. The results of the election were announced in assembly and Dr. Kester gave the boys, both of them, a huge hug to show his congratulations. It was a wonderful way to learn the meaning of equality. Dr. Kester had taught me a deep truth. I would never forget it.

When I was alone all I could do was hope that it would remain the same. Could I hope for that? I ploughed into the books for my grade nine exams. Hope would not be enough. I wanted to give myself every possible chance of success. The results came back. Mr. Dicks called me to his office.

Susanne, you have done a good job, he said. I had passed grade nine with 91 percent. The next year I would take a course of study that would lead to a full ten papers in grade thirteen.

I wished that the summer wasn't as long as it was. It was difficult to be excited about the summer holidays as the other kids were – there would be no cottages and dances and swimming and fun jobs for me. There would just be the garden and the radio, my books and my parents and anticipation about September.

But the success that I was enjoying at school came home with me, if only just a little bit. That summer I was given more responsibilities. I helped in the kitchen and I was allowed to dress myself. I missed school but the months passed quietly and relatively happily in the summer sun and the green garden.

I was in grade ten!

I had three more subjects but my work load, although really doubled, seemed to be ten times what it had been. It was the amount of mechanical work that gave me the trouble, that and the more frenzied and hurried feeling that was created by the lack of spare time. Whereas once I had had time to get to classes, now I had none. And I couldn't tuck my books under an arm as the others did and run through the halls, through the miles and miles (or so it seemed) of locker-covered corridors to the next class. I urged my muscles, my spastic legs, to make the journey more speedily but they couldn't hear, or they wouldn't listen. I arrived at most classes late and exhausted by this demanding expense of energy, almost too tired to lift my pencil and take down the notes that all the other students scribbled with their fast hands.

The material was no harder to understand; it was just a question of being able to find the time to think about it and learn it. There was no spare time. Every second was devoted to the almost futile task of staying up to date with my notes. I would work in my infrequent empty periods, during lunch hours, after school and after supper. The radio could no longer be my leisurely companion; I was always tired, my muscles were made even more unruly by the constant physical pressures. I became more nervous; sometimes I was barely able to eat. This anxiety and my drive to succeed wore on me; my marks fell, my spirit fell, my enthusiasm lagged to the constant worry of defeat.

And then I found a solution. I developed my own very workable shorthand system. It was simple enough that my fellow students could understand it. It helped me to overcome the odds enough for school to regain the glamour that it had been fast losing. My marks went up, and my spirit rose with them. I had competitors, Joe and Ernie. How I loved to beat them on a test, and how I worked so that I would stand in front of them in the finals.

The school authorities were very fair in evaluating me. I wrote as much as I could of the normal written examination and then

I was given a supplementary oral exam as well. I was a well-examined student. I had to work hard and I loved it.

My marks improved through grades ten and eleven and finally I stood in the top ten in the entire school in grade twelve. I beat Joe and Ernie that year.

At home things had been improving. My parents were beginning to accept my abilities, to question their previous opinions about the nature of their poor sick girl. But it was difficult for them, and when things went wrong I was the easiest target. Things did go wrong.

The factory where my father was employed went bankrupt. He was out of work, home brooding, almost insane from the lack of activity. Mother was working. It seemed that all his recriminations were directed to me on those summer days. There was no escape but to the state of sickness and worry that mirrored his own. I lost my appetite completely, broke out in a severe rash caused no doubt by the nervous imbalance of my system and a lack of nourishment. I was finally taken to the family doctor but the consultation seemed more devoted to his recriminations. Did I deserve the medical aid he was administering? I had done so well in school – me, sickly, spastic Susanne Moss. And his nephew George had failed.

My mother did not escape that summer without some outside pressure. Most of her fellow workers had children who were my classmates and friends. She would be questioned about how I could write and even give notes to the other students or help those who were having trouble that I could straighten out. Mother was so confused by all these questions.

She was asked how could such a sick girl, such a shame, be able to do this. She never bothered to find the answers to the questions. She couldn't cope with the ridicule.

Instead, when school reopened I was forbidden to go on the bus. I would either be taken or take a taxi. She would not allow my friends in the house. I could not leave the house; I had to come home right after school. She would not have these women talking about her daughter. No, the shame had gone far enough – it would go no farther.

Father's factory reopened under new management in late August. He went back to work; I went into grade thirteen. My friends could only be visited within the few hours of the school day. Dr. Kester had left to take a better job in the States; Mr. Dicks had to leave because of poor health. My world was crumbling.

The grade twelve graduation ceremonies were scheduled in the fall on my grade thirteen year. I looked forward to the event, and envisaged the occasion with excitement and like the other girls asked my mother to help me buy a gown. She wasn't sure that the school officials would want one who was sick at the ceremony, and she postponed the purchase until she was assured that I would be welcomed.

Our search for the appropriate attire for the event led to the first hostile reaction from the outside world in many years.

My mother and I were in the most expensive ladies' store in the town, eyeing the beauty of the evening dresses, the formal lines, the pretty bows, when a saleswoman asked if she could help. My mother told her of my need for a graduation gown. The woman, haughty in disbelief, surveyed me, my twitching muscles.

Oh, she was quite certain that this store could not outfit me. She suggested that we continue our search in another store, of much poorer quality.

I shrugged off this woman's rudeness as an isolated incident. I was, after all, a grade twelve graduate; only the very ignorant and mean would treat me in such a degrading manner.

We finally found a dress. Mother went alone and bought the gown I needed. Dr. Kester made the trip to the graduation especially to see me. The Board of Education members made a big fuss over my achievement. It was a wonderful night. I thought my heart would pop with pride as I walked up across the stage to receive my diploma. My friends and classmates were there. They all stood and cheered as the chairman handed me that wonderful piece of paper. I hoped my parents would feel some of this pride, that they could see that I was not a shame but a responsible student who had worked hard against severe odds and had earned the respect and the accolades that the gathering had given me.

I think that they were impressed. We drove home that night in a close to festive mood. I was tired and as happy as I had ever been; my parents were confused and yet I think happy as well. Before I said goodnight, my father turned to me, his brow creased in concentration as if he had been revising all the thoughts he had felt about me previously.

You know, Susanne, he said, with all those big shots so enthusiastic about you, you won't have a bad time getting along in life.

I think I smiled and said goodnight.

I had to write the departmental examinations in grade thirteen just like everyone else. I wrote as much as I could. My hands were so sore and my muscles were so exhausted after each paper that I thought it would be impossible to take the next one. But somehow I did.

The marks returned. I had passed, but my marks had dropped appreciably. I worried that they would not be good enough to get me to university, but I made the application anyway. I was accepted at Duncan University at Mooreland, a school where Dr. Kester had many friends. Yes, I was going to university. Me, Susanne Moss, I was going to university. I wondered about all those ignorant people who had asked about the sick little girl, who had with fiendish concern counselled my parents on the arts of murdering such a burden. But they didn't matter anymore. I had worked long and hard and cried and worked even harder and now I was going to university. I had the letter. "The Board of Governors is pleased to announce that you have been accepted to Duncan University." Wasn't anything possible?

Of course my mother was concerned at the prospects of my going away to school. I think she still had visions of my being tortured if I was taken away from her, but my father was, in some ways, almost as excited as I was.

I wrote requesting an appointment for a Saturday so that both my parents could make the trip and see the school. Then one glorious day in early August, we were off to Mooreland.

We toured the small campus before our appointment with the dean. We walked through the small gardens, the flowers brilliant in the warm August sun. I delighted in the new shining buildings, and I saw the lecture rooms, the library, the cafeteria, and imagined the next four years with growing hope. It would be so meaningful, to learn in these rooms, to read these books, to discuss and laugh in the comfortable cafeteria. I envisaged sitting with friends in the spring, under the newly budding trees, overlooking the lake out behind the residence, eagerly discussing all that we had learned the previous year, anxious about the coming examinations.

I took my father's hand as we made our visit. I watched my mother's face, the happy expression. Perhaps it would be a new phase in our relationship. I thanked them.

Miss Green, the dean of women, met us in her office at the appointed hour. She was gracious, and charming. I thought her dress a little inappropriate for an elderly woman of her position. I turned to my mother; she obviously thought the same as I – the dress was too tight and a little short. But I guessed that was the way a dean of women dressed. This was, after all, very new to both of us.

The graciousness and charm turned a little cool after she asked why we had asked for a Saturday appointment and was told that my parents both worked. I wondered what that had to do with anything, but her attitude seemed to imply that it did. I decided that I didn't like Miss Green but thought it in my best interests not to allow this sentiment to become obvious.

In the course of our discussion I mentioned the fact that my marks had dropped drastically in the grade thirteen departmentals and asked what kind of arrangements could be worked out to avoid this same occurrence at Duncan. Miss Green had already talked to the dean about the matter. Through consultation, the two deans and the registrar had decided that I would be able to dictate my exams.

But, she said, it must be understood that this arrangement is not the usual practice. Never in the past has this been granted. Blind students have been allowed to type their exams, but never has there been a case where dictation was allowed.

I must be very, very thankful, she explained, and added that she thought it would be a good idea if I purchased a typewriter and learned to type.

My father said that he would buy me a typewriter immediately. Miss Green told us about the fine and gifted people who were associated with Duncan, both as students and staff. She finished; the interview ended.

My mother and father both seemed pleased with the visit to Duncan, with the cleanliness of the residences and the person of Miss Green. But I didn't. I sat silent in the back seat during the trip home. I listened to my parents discuss the day while a growing gloom darkened all the enthusiasm that I had felt about university while it was far away. I didn't know just exactly why but there was something wrong with the place. All I could do for the rest of the month before the opening of classes was to hope that my intuition had been incorrect, to pray that it would be a good place, and that life would continue in the way that I had grown to expect it would and should.

It was a difficult feeling to overcome. I kept thinking of the manner in which Miss Green addressed me, her cool attitude towards my parents because they both had to work. But was that really fair, to judge an entire university, the times I would have there, the treatment I would receive, just from one person? No, it wasn't fair, it wasn't right. Or was it?

The day before I was to leave for school, I received a telegram:

> I REGRET TO INFORM YOU THAT THE ACCEPTANCE OF YOUR APPLICATION WAS A MISTAKE STOP
>
> REGISTRAR.

No, no, this had to be an error. I had been there, I had spoken to the dean of women. She was expecting me. I rushed through a call to Dr. Kester, demanded that his secretary interrupt his meeting, then cried through the cables of the Bell System on the injustices of the world. He was almost as shaken by this communication as I was, but assured me that he would speak to Dean Elder immediately and straighten out the obvious mistake.

Another telegram arrived at three o'clock the same afternoon. Ah yes, there had been a serious mistake.

I left for Duncan the next day. Who, I wondered, was making the mistakes?

I was somewhat surprised by the warm reception I received at Duncan. How could I expect them to be so receptive after the telegram episode of the previous day? But they seemed genuinely glad to see me, even Miss Green, the same smile on top of the same dress, or was it another of the same skimpy cut? Dean Elder was distinguished and patronly, his graying temples, his clammy handshake. The bespectacled registrar in his best suit was wearing his introduction smile.

WELCOME TO DUNCAN

There was my big sister Rozanne, so helpful and knowing. If all the students were like her, Duncan would be a fine place. Rozanne showed me the school in a new light. It was a busy day with people and trunks and waves from across lawns and warm handshakes that said "I'm glad you are back." And noisy residences, gossipy conversation, the latest news of the professors, who to take classes from and who to avoid, talk about the football team and the first dance. I had never been to a football game or a dance. But I would. I was a student of Duncan University now.

Classes started with a festive frivolity that I found somewhat confusing after my high school experience and my expectations about the serious nature of a university education. There were line ups in the bookstore, more gossip about the newest of the romances on campus. I wondered why I was the only person in the residence library most evenings.

And then two weeks into the term Miss Green called me to her office. I thought surely she was going to congratulate me on the attitude I had taken towards my work at Duncan. I was working even harder than I had during high school; I never missed classes and asked questions of the teachers whenever I was puzzled. In fact I was quite certain that no one could fault my behaviour or attitude. But I must have been wrong; this visit to Miss Green was the first in a series of lectures. Subject: Susanne Moss was unappreciative of the opportunity that Duncan had given her; she must be more humble, more aware of the fine Christian tradition of the school and the prestige of the institution.

These were not discussions. I was never allowed a word although an apology was always expected; I was expected to apologize for living.

Duncan became so lonely after that. I had no friends other than Rozanne, and she was a senior student and had her work and her friends. It was difficult to expect her company all the time. There were my studies, but they became lonely without the sharing of problems and the discussions that had been part of high school. In desperation I turned to the Anglican club, the largest club on campus. Wasn't the church supposed to offer love to all? I wanted comfort, friendship, involvement.

My association with the church afforded a great deal of comfort through the year. I liked the ceremony of the services, the words of the minister; but there was so much that I asked the church to do. Was it reasonable of me to ask that it make life at Duncan tolerable? It had so much to overcome.

Most nights I went to bed early because of exhaustion, but since the residence walls were thin and the discipline in the place was non-existent, it was impossible to sleep. My roommates were typical of the girls in the residence. They were away from home for the first time and school was easy. They could devote their time to preening, hairdressing, and idle gossip about the boys and their dates. I could have forgiven them this; – it was their world, quite alien to mine – but I couldn't accept their lack of consideration. I couldn't count the number of times that they awakened me after a late night, the number of conversations I listened to about sex, the times they would leave me out of anything else they were doing. I remember overhearing them one night.

It's too bad that Susanne is such a square.

Yeah, the only thing she's interested in is working.

But they were wrong. I wanted to go to the parties, to laugh with friends, at least in the beginning.

I retreated to my books. I struggled through each day as both an outcast and an oddity. There were never words of encouragement – only the frequent and humiliating interviews with Miss Green.

I searched for the fine qualities of the staff that the dean of women was always touting but found only mediocracy in their abilities and a general disregard for the academic stimulation of their students. I sought out-of-class contact with these men, but found only disdain. How could these people be in charge of the education of the students? And yet they were. These were the fine Christian staff members of this august university, these men who lectured from the textbooks, or spent their lecture time discussing unassociated aspects of their lives, doing anything but stimulating, teaching, or even interesting the bored and unappreciative students.

It was little wonder that the majority of the students ignored their school work, spent their time dating and partying rather than pursuing their education. But there was nothing for me to do.

I sought involvement with what clubs were offered. I became more involved with the Anglican club. I kept hoping that something would happen to make life more meaningful. Perhaps, I thought, I was just homesick and things were getting to me more than they would when this state had passed. But when my parents made their monthly visits I knew that I could never be homesick. I had passed that contact with home and family.

By Christmas I knew that I would not be returning the following year, that I must make the best of the year I would have at Duncan and then go on to something else. It is painful when one finally realizes the futility of dreams and ambitions, when it becomes all too clear that the path that was chosen was wrong.

But who was wrong?

There was a Christmas dinner in the residence. All the girls were required to have dates drawn by lot. I was forced into that alien world, the world of Betty and Joan, and most of the students; roses and make-up, excitement and anxiety. I went to the dinner, and surprisingly had a very good time. But when the dance was about to start, my date asked if he could be excused from the remainder of the evening. He would like to pick up his girl friend.

Of course.

I spent the night alone in the library. I stared at the rows and rows of books, all that knowledge that I once hoped would be mine during my years at university – years of opportunity when I could show my industry, rise above the poverty and ignorance of my upbringing. I believed that once. But it wasn't true. It wasn't true if you could never be accepted outside the lecture halls, if you couldn't go to a dance, if you didn't have a boyfriend and share in the gossip and tell of your romantic experiences. That was just as important, maybe more important.

No, I didn't belong. The university authorities reversed their promise and decided that since I had a typewriter I would be required to type my Christmas exams rather than dictate them. I pleaded with the registrar and Miss Green. I couldn't even type my essays. But they were quite firm. A schedule was issued. I was to report to various rooms on mornings of my exams and bring my typewriter. I lugged it all over the university that week, the twenty pounds made more heavy by the uselessness of my appearance. I could never pass this way, not with my slow spastic two fingers jerking to the constant passing of each precious second. I was given no extra time. What was the use of studying, why did I even know what I did? I couldn't possibly pass if I had three times the amount of time allotted.

When the results were released I was not surprised that I had failed, but to add to the injustices of the procedure, I had been marked for my typing mistakes as well. I made representation to the dean, to the registrar. Everyone was too busy to see me. So many questions were left unanswered when I went home for the holidays.

My entire body, my mind, my will to live had been numbed by those four months. At home it was no better; my parents boasted about the sacrifices they were making so that I could go to university. They ignored my statements about the place, discounted my unhappiness, treated me once again like the "poor sick thing."

I returned in January to the coldness, made more severe by the winter months. There was a new psychology club that eased some of the boredom and there was still the church, gaining more and more of my time. There was always the loneliness, the sense of futility, the noisy residence and the ostracism of my class and roommates.

Spring arrived, the grass grew green, the boys played baseball, the libraries filled. It was almost over. When the final examination schedule was posted, I asked that I be allowed to dictate my exams. But the same procedure would be followed; I did not protest.

I failed. I went home to the recriminations of my parents. They were confused. How could I have wasted all that money, they asked. But they never listened to my answers.

My father went to see the dean, demanded that I be permitted to repeat the year, protested the waste of his money. Dean Elder said nothing, only that Susanne had failed and the university could not allow her to return.

Slowly and bitterly my father concurred with me. He cursed the injustices of the English society, accused the rich of plotting to keep the poor uneducated. His bitterness grew through that summer, while mine waned. The nightmare had ended for me but my father made plans: I would work on my typing and get a job as a stenographer like daughters of his friends.

I laughed at such counselling. I could never be a stenographer, but it didn't matter, not really. All that mattered was that I get away, find a job, and try to forget my year at Duncan. All the world couldn't be that bad.

Part II

Part II

Five years later I knew a little better. I sat waiting in the reception room of the Toronto Rehabilitation Centre. I stared at the clock on the wall – the white face and the sweeping second hand. The uncomfortable wooden chair dug into my twitching body. People came and went but ignored me. I sat and watched the clock. What was time? It seemed to me that morning only a period of frustration and loneliness – I sat waiting.

I had struggled with the padlock on the gate that surrounded my garden too many times. Lost five years – five years lost in spastic muscles and a key that I could not make fit the rusted cheap lock. Behind it my tormented parents had retreated from their shame, had neglected their simmering pots for the prepared spaghetti and beans that mushed from mechanically opened tins. They never smiled above their cups of coffee and would sometimes leave me unnoticed as I sat in the lonely living room with the silent broken radio and a stack of books from the library.

There had been times during those five years when I too could retreat, hide behind a red covered book jacket and ignore what was becoming clear – the slamming doors, the secretaries who said that their bosses were out of town while they sat behind glass partitions.

Yes, I had started to look for work. I had started with employment agencies but found that my education had done very little to train me for an office position. The employment counsellors, at least those who would see me, took one look at my scrawling and slow writing, a quick glance at my application sheet and the courses that I had taken in high school, and dismissed me.

We can't find you a position. I'm sorry.

I spent lonely nights sitting in the living room. The chairs were becoming worn looking, the wallpaper was yellowing, the silence from my parents, a doorway away, was errie.

Occasionally my father had asked about the progress of my typing.

Susanne, practise your typing, he would yell through the walls.

But why? The books could last forever I sometimes thought.

There was my handicap pension, a bed, and the spaghetti that mushed from tins.

Friends had tried to help me fill the time; they had attempted to shield me from the abuse that always surrounded me. They had encouraged me to join the Young People's group at the church and I had been excited by the stimulation such contact afforded. Even the church seemed friendly on those Wednesday evenings – the smell of fresh floor wax on the yellow linoleum in the basement Sunday school room, the large table in the kitchen and the cups of steaming coffee, egg salad sandwiches, and butter tarts. I was a member of a group again, the way I had been in high school.

But finally nothing could help. The lonely Sunday morning walks, my slow retreat down the front stone steps of the church – the sunlight and whispered jeers had overridden my enthusiasm. I could not even feel welcome in the dark oak pews of a church. I was not welcome. Not in church, not in offices. My twitching muscles repulsed people when I tried to move toward them with a greeting, with a question. I stood alone, I walked alone and I had returned alone to the padlock and the neglected garden, weedy and stubbled through five springs and summers, covered with fall dead leaves, buried in five winters of grey snow.

And now, five years after I had returned home from Duncan, I sat in the stark waiting room of the Toronto Rehabilitation Centre. I thought back as the clock on the wall counted the past minutes. I thought about the past, about my parents' threats, the three months somewhere in those years when I had remained in my bed, afraid for my life. I recalled, over and over again, my mother waving the knife at me. I had tried to reason with them.

Mother, there is no reason for you not to go to Lilian's wedding.

But they could not hear. The inflicted shame of my handicap still too heavy.

Shut up or I will kill you, she said.

Why can't you accept me for what I am?

Shut up, my father yelled.

I stepped back, I saw my mother's head in front of the dirty kitchen window. She wore a loose-fitting brown dress, soiled on the front, and a black moth-eaten cardigan sweater. She waved the knife in her right hand; bread crumbs fell from the blade. My father sat at the table in front of a half-eaten plate of pork and beans. They both turned their heads to look at me, but their eyes could not see. I saw. I saw two pairs of eyes, clouded by induced hate and disappointment. They could not go to Lilian's wedding. I really believed that they would kill me. I really believed that I would never escape their house, would perish within those decaying walls and be buried in the neglected garden, never having achieved any kind of job or independence.

I had rushed to my room in panic. I grabbed the worn wood bannister with both hands to aid my slow legs. I pulled myself as fast as I could to escape. I stumbled once on one of the loose rubber mats that protected the stairs. Did I really hear my mother coming after me or was it imagination? I didn't turn around to look. I never wanted to turn around and look at those years in that house. I had to leave.

The clock in the reception room wall had moved through two hours since I had arrived that morning. There were no magazines and the room was uncomfortable. Occasionally the receptionist would disappear behind a door and return with a cup of coffee. People walked in and identified themselves and left me alone with the clock and my memories.

I had waited a long time. My minister had helped a great deal in arranging this appointment. It had seemed a reasonable place to go after the failure at the provincial Welfare Office, after the disappointment with the unemployment people.

I could hear muffled conversation from behind doors; occasionally a telephone would ring. I sat and waited. I thought about all the waiting I had done, about how long it had taken to get an appointment with the provincial Welfare Office in Toronto and that morning when one of the social workers had taken me to the Crippled Civilian Headquarters.

I had been so full of hope the afternoon before. I had gone shopping. I had wandered the downtown area and imagined that it had always been there, that I had always been in Toronto. I would be, and Eaton's and Simpsons would be just a subway ride away and the museum and the movie theatres, libraries, a new church where people would not whisper and jeer. Everything had seemed possible that afternoon. That night I went to sleep with new dreams.

And in the morning a woman from the Welfare Office had met me promptly at nine o'clock and driven me to the Crippled Civilian Headquarters. But the city gradually lost the grace of the previous afternoon; the cleanliness had vanished by the time we had reached our destination. A dilapidated building, hardly standing it seemed, awaited our arrival.

An unoiled door opened into a long dark hallway; chipped gray paint covered the unstable bricks that formed the passage. The floor groaned as we walked towards the elevator cage. I said nothing, the woman seemed not to notice the disrepair of the building. The elevator stopped on the second floor, the door opened. I caught a glimpse of the rows and rows of small wooden benches, with wheelchairs in evidence at most of the poorly lit cubicles. The elevator continued its climb, I tried to ignore the unsafe noises of the ascent, but was relieved when we got off at the next floor, a copy of the first, and proceeded to the director's office.

Mr. Mann's office had seemed even more lavish than it was beside the squalor of the rest of the building. I stared in disbelief at the brightly polished floor, the new colourful drapes, the shining office equipment.

He greeted me with little enthusiasm, and voiced his intentions to test my physical abilities to determine what sort of job I could fill in his operations. I asked if he planned to have me work on the second floor, amongst the filth and bad lighting, weaving baskets, or spending my day on simple needlework.

Why, of course.

No, no; I had not fallen that far. I would escape my family, but never to be interned in a different cage. I would not be shut away from sunlight and self-respect, dabbling away at such a demeaning occupation, subservient to those who had created this factory for society's rejects. There had to be something else and I had gambled on just that hope when I told them, the two of them, that I would not work in such a place.

That had been two years before. I had been waiting for two years, and now another three hours in the Rehabilitation Centre. I was exhausted by the effort that it had taken to control my steady sitting position. I was tired of waiting.

The receptionist came towards me.

The doctor is ready to give you your medical examination now, Miss Moss. This way, please. Through the mysterious door that I had watched people go and come from for three hours.

I was escorted to another room just as stark, attended by a doctor with expressionless eyes, with probing fingers. Occasionally he would mumble over his shoulder to the disinterested nurse who was keeping notes.

Spastic C.P., he said

What's that? I asked.

What do you mean what's that? He seemed almost amused.

What's Spastic C.P.?

The disinterested expression gave way to one of disbelief. He addressed me for the first time.

Don't you know what's wrong with you?

No. I've always been told I was sick, that's all, just sick.

He helped me up from the examination table and invited me into his office. I was very tired and very tense, my muscles seemed more alien than they usually did. I could not relax. The doctor helped me into a chair.

You have spastic cerebral palsy.

I had only read the words. They had never meant anything to me, but he went on to explain the brain injury involved and some of my symptoms. He seemed very reluctant to talk about what could be done to help me. He had another appointment he said. The nurse reappeared to escort me to another room.

Thank you, doctor. He didn't reply; I guess he didn't hear me.

The other room was another waiting room. It had two chairs and a desk. It didn't have a clock.

Five weeks later I sat in a room very similar; it may even have been the same room. The walls, all the walls, had the same nondescript colour, a sort of browny-yellowy-white, aged and dirty. There was an old desk and chairs that wobbled. There had been five weeks of similar rooms and wobbling chairs. I had moved from occupation to occupation with the schedule that had been arranged. I was being tested, graded, and judged so that someone could decide what kind of occupation I could physically handle.

Their only concern was to determine my physical capabilities. I tried very hard to be co-operative and pleasant with the banalities that I had to put up with. I did not find my tasks terribly difficult – they were like most physical problems that I had encountered: the more I worked at them, the more familiar my muscles became with the routine and movements involved and the more able I was to achieve some sort of success. Through the five weeks I did progress. I became more able to manoeuvre sheets of paper in the inky and dusty old printing press. I stapled papers together. One week I used an electric typewriter; it was very frustrating because of the light touch involved and my inability to rest my fingers on the keys without engaging the mechanism. In another room, in another week, they gave me an adding machine and endless columns of figures. There was a certain amount of satisfaction during this exercise. I didn't mind pushing the numbered buttons, cranking the sticky arm on the side of the machine, ripping off of the roll of white paper, and comparing the exactness of my answer beside the answer that I had determined more quickly by adding the way I was taught in school.

I was not very good in many of these tests, but there was one that I had excelled at, probably because I had found it so simple compared with my outside pursuits at the time. One of the efficient and cool workers would give me a pair of potholders and with precise and rather perfunctorary instructions and pencilled lines, have me sew lines, or sometimes circles in the material. At the time, during my lonely evenings in my room at the YWCA, I was starting to do church embroidery, an interest and occupation that certainly required far more skill and precision than the menial task of putting thread into a lined linen potholder. I was always amused by the reaction that I received from the potholder test. I suppose it was astonishing to note the slow and laboured work that I did at a typewriter beside the quick and efficient sewing that I exhibited in the potholder room.

But there was never any encouragement. I had a feeling that I was always being watched, perhaps charted and graded and inspected, but I could find no reason for the terse and precise instructions. I was eager to learn, but learning could not be spontaneous in such a place. I began to wonder why I had come to the centre, why each day I made the lonely bus journey, with the stares of curiosity and the whispered comments, only to be left frustrated and alone in one of the many small rooms with the wobbly chairs.

There had only been one woman in the entire centre who treated me with any respect whatsoever and indeed seemed eager and able to help me. Her room had a window. Sunshine shone through the dirty glass, gaily picking up specks of dust that danced through the lines of sunlight to her dark wood desk with the tape recorder. In my first meeting she had just talked to me. I hadn't known why – it was unusual for anyone just to sit down and talk to me. She asked me what I hoped to do with my education and about how I liked Toronto and living at the Y. After fifteen minutes or so she pulled her tape recorder out from behind the desk and played it back to me.

I heard her ask a question.

Then I heard an agonizing, certainly almost undistinguishable voice answer in what might have been English, but that was open to question. The voice squeeked and blurred. I listened very carefully, not really knowing what was going on, what this was all about, and then suddenly I caught a word and realized rather embarrassingly that the voice was mine, unoiled and garbled.

I was shocked. Why hadn't anybody ever demonstrated or at least told me about this very crucial impediment before? I had met with employment counsellors, I had been interviewed by various agencies for the handicapped, and never once had I been advised to take speech therapy. It seemed, all of a sudden, little wonder that I had so much trouble in securing a job. It was very difficult for people to understand what I was saying.

I met with the speech therapist every day for my last three weeks at the centre. In the room with the sunlight, the tape recorder, and her patient smiling face; I exercised my dormant tongue, stretched my lips and facial muscles, and made conscious efforts to slow my speech. I made progress, and she started me on a program that I no doubt would have continued had it not been for my final meeting in the centre.

In the final week, the potholders having been all finished, they took some tests that were intelligence oriented and not simply of a physical nature. For these I sat behind the desks. The chairs did not wobble as much as the chairs that faced the desks.

I had finished my first work of church embroidery and sold it to the Anglican Bookshop. I was encouraged to continue this line of work and had been gaining friends and assistance towards this end. I was growing tired and questioned the point of my time at the centre. The walls were growing dingier and only the speech therapist smiled at me; the others were too interested in the sheet of paper that they studied and on which they pencilled my progress.

The five weeks were finally ended and once again I waited in a room. Again there was a clock, a second hand sweeping away minutes in a steady arc. I was going to be given the results of my tests, steps would be recommended as to what and where to go in order to secure employment. Again the chair wobbled, one leg rested in the dusty air of the room. There was no window and no sunlight. A man and a woman entered.

The man looked down at the folder in front of him. The woman walked around my chair and stood against the wall to my left. I sat and waited for their advice.

Miss Moss, your I.Q. is above average. But . . .

But what?

But your physical incapabilities lead us to the unpleasant conclusion that you will never be able to work. Fortunately, there is always your pension and you could return to your parents.

The second hand stopped. I didn't hear what the man was saying. I stared at him but he turned away. My spasm increased, my hands and legs shook more fiercely than I could ever remember.

I screamed. No. How could this be true. I had paid money, wasted time. For what? To be told that I could never work. I had just sold some work to the Anglican Bookshop.

I demanded to see the director of the centre. Something was wrong. I screamed again. More people rushed into the small room. I threatened to expose the place as a sham, these people as corrupt merchants of hope.

I was hysterical. Fortunately one of the women administrators got me out of the building to a quiet cup of coffee. I calmed down and told her about what had been said and how I had been thinking about going into the field of church embroidery. She persuaded me to contact a Mr. Allison at the March of Dimes Workshop.

I received both funds and encouragement from Mr. Allison at the March of Dimes. That, and a happier view of conditions in which some handicapped individuals worked; fluorescent lighting and windows did wonders to make a place seem cheerier than the decrepit second floor at the Crippled Civilian Headquarters Workshop. Mr. Allison seemed an oddity at first glance; he smiled and seemed genuinely interested in my prospects and ambitions. He did not keep his head buried in a statistics sheet or keep me waiting in a room with a clock and bare walls.

I had made more contacts in the field and had learned that because of a lack of qualified people Canada was forced to import close to a hundred thousand dollars of church embroidery every year. People were helping me and I sold vestments to young divinity students who could not afford the more expensive prices of others' goods.

Of course, I needed this help. I did enjoy sitting over my small desk in my room at the Y struggling with the fine detail of the work, forcing my hands to obey the precise detailed moves that were necessary, and I was achieving better and better quality, but there were certain steps that my contacts could not help me with, that seemed too complicated to copy from material that was lent to me. As in all things I did not want to have to rely on a second-rate skill and the perverse nature of people who might buy my goods because I was handicapped. My friends understood this and the Canon at my new church, St. Radegund's, made an appointment for me with the top authority in the field, a nun who lived in and oversaw the embroidery operations at an Anglican convent outside of Toronto. I was assured of her assistance and even perhaps of some extra work as it was general knowledge that the sisters could not fill all the orders they received.

I had to take a bus that morning on a cold January day, dark and wintry at six-thirty. Tiny snow flakes filled the morning air and mixed with the exhaust of the buses that roared in and out of the terminal at Bay and Dundas. I was tired and nervous, not used to getting up so early in the morning. The stares that I received from the transients in the coffee shop made me even more uncomfortable. I was glad when my bus was called and I could, although awkwardly, retreat to the back of the bus and hide from the stares in the anonymity of the cold double seat. My appointment had been arranged for quite early so that I would not interrupt the nun during her heavy schedule. I was just happy to be able to meet her and did not make any objections to the time. I had with me some of my work and some borrowed work which had stitching that I needed help with.

It was a slow trip through the waking city. Cars moved slowly through the cold and flying snow and clogged the traffic. When the bus stopped to pick up travellers, the January wind swept through the open doors. The compartment never warmed quite enough before the bus would stop and winter would enter again.

The day grew lighter but the snow fell heavier. I did not know this part of the country. I sat against the window with my coat closed around me and watched the icy countryside until finally the bus stopped at a small restaurant in a very small town. That was a far as the bus would take me. I got up to get off. I grabbed my satchel with the embroidery, gathered my scarf and hat. I was still very cold and moved slowly, my spasm made worse with the cold. The bus driver yelled back.

Hurry up, lady.

The door was open, waiting for me. I tried to hurry. I was just almost to the door when it closed.

I yelled for him to let me out.

Finally one of the passengers saw that I was handicapped and helped me. He helped me down the icy black steps and left me on the lonely snowy sidewalk in a town whose name I had only heard the morning before. The bus moved away, its black exhaust wrapped its choking warmth around me.

I went into the restaurant and asked about a taxi. The convent was almost a mile away, a deserted retreat that I had been told was simply lovely in the summer, with beautiful gardens and friendly people. The man behind the counter was Chinese, a cigarette dangled from his lips as he leaned over his coffee and newspaper. A long ash dropped into the coffee that he had spilled in the saucer. I asked him if there was some way that I could get to the convent, a taxi or perhaps a local bus.

Sorry, lady. You like coffee?

I was already late for my appointment time, delayed by the slow progress of the bus. I asked what direction the convent was, and the man very kindly drew me a map. He said that it was just a half a mile.

I thanked him and left the warmth of the restaurant and started to walk. Occasionally I would stop and turn my head away from the wind and check my progress on the map that the man had drawn me. It took me forty-five minutes to reach the convent, through the front gates and up the drive to the large wooden door. I was an hour late for my appointment.

I reached for the large black iron door knocker. My hands were so cold I had to make several attempts to grab it. I finally managed and knocked as hard as I could. I stood and waited for some reply. I knocked again and waited again.

I hear the lock, the bolt inside, and then an eye peeped through the cracked opening followed by a voice.

What do you want?

I told her about my appointment and why I had been delayed. I'm sorry but I thought perhaps the sister could see me anyway when I have already come all this way.

I'll see, replied the voice. The door slammed. I stood waiting on the snowy doorstep. The wind seemed to get stronger and colder as it attacked me in front of the big wooden door.

You can come in. She escorted me through the front halls to a waiting room, its walls lined with bookcases with very few books. Wait, she said and left.

I waited and tried to warm myself, but the room seemed cold and I left my coat on. My spasm was bad, worsened no doubt by the chill in my bones. I sat and watched the doorway and waited for the sister who was an embroidery expert and a nun in the Anglican Church. I waited and wished that I could have a cup of coffee, that I had sat and talked to the helpful Chinese man in the little restaurant and warmed myself somewhat before starting my hike through the slippery country roads.

Finally a nun entered the room. I got up to meet her and she backed away from my approach.

Good morning, I'm Susanne Moss. Canon Coalier made an appointment for me.

What's wrong with you? she said.

I'm cold so I didn't take my coat off.

No, you're shaking so much and your voice.

I have cerebral palsy.

Oh.

Could I show you some of my embroidery?

I don't have time to see you. I think you should go. We are very busy here at the convent. There are so many orders for our work.

Are there any I could fill? I asked. I was told that perhaps there would be and I do need the work.

No. no. There is just enough work for us. I think you should go.

She left the room. She hurried, her black gown flew from her body as she turned left at the doorway.

I put my scarf back on and made my way through the halls, between the hanging tapestry, the scenes of gardens and saints. I had trouble opening the door, the wind made it heavier.

I walked back the way I came, back to the restaurant. Cars slowed and the drivers looked at me. It was an easier walk but it was more agonizing. The wind was behind me, pushing me away from the convent.

The Chinese man was still behind the counter in the restaurant. More ashes had fallen into his coffee saucer. He poured me a cup of coffee and we sat and talked in the deserted little restaurant until the bus from Toronto came and returned me to my room at the Y and my embroidery work which no longer seemed so exciting.

My church embroidery venture faded throughout the remainder of that year. It was finally just too tedious, too difficult to sit and control my hands when I was only making samples that were never sold. Many friends helped but I could not compete in the high salesmanship end of the operation. I had tried; I had set out my goods on a table in rooms with the major suppliers. When it was discovered that the work was mine, I received no orders. The vestments I sold to the divinity students took too much time for too little money, and I finally had to admit the futility of the situation.

I got a box, and on a rainy afternoon in September I cleaned my room at the Y of all the evidence that I had been involved with the demanding field of church embroidery.

I knew there would always be demands, however. I would not allow this setback to mean defeat, and return to my parents and the continual boredom and fear of a life in their home.

I started instead to make dresses for people I knew, people who could not afford the established dressmakers and who could not buy their clothes off the rack. It was not a new thing for me. I had been making my own clothes for a number of years and had received compliments on them. Some of the ladies at the church were very willing to order goods from me on a trial basis. And with the loan of a portable sewing machine, I made a dress for one of these women which so impressed her that she decided to help further by soliciting aid from others in the church.

To this end, a dinner party was arranged, and on a glorious fall evening I was picked up at the Y and driven to the Raymonds' house in Rosedale.

I had never driven in a Cadillac before, had never sunk into the deep-piled back seat, and laughed with the warm comfort that such an evening projected. We drove slowly through the winding oak and maple lined streets while the Nelsons pointed out some of the magnificient houses and what brief history they knew of the occupants. We finally drove into the winding gravel driveway of the Raymonds.

Their house was certainly the match of any. The grass still seemed green through the fallen leaves, and the gardens showed deep rich brown earth and surrounded the white stone of the house. The setting sun played with the trees and danced over the house and the cars in the drive. It gave a comfort and friendliness to the place. I was sure that it would be a happy evening. Mr. Nelson helped me out of the car and I took his arm as he escorted me to the front door.

The Raymonds were indeed very gracious hosts. The solid splendour and luxuriousness of their house wrapped itself around the guests. The pictures that hung in the living room were bright and vivid and seemed to demand smiles. The yellows and blues of the decor, the grey-haired handsomeness of the host and the charm of the hostess all played as one, combining to intone warmth and a good-naturedness that I had never experienced in a gathering.

I sat and drank sherry in a large tumbler and did not feel

embarrassed by my necessity to use such a glass. I talked with some of the people whom I had met but briefly outside of St. Radegund's on Sunday mornings. They had seemed occupied on these occasions but they were intently interested with me this evening. Laughter rose from parts of the room, it mixed with the tinkling of ice cubes and the men's jokes about football. The servers, two women in black dresses with white starched collars and sleeves, mingled with sterling silver trays heaped with hot and cold hors d'oeuvres. One of these women started to make a fuss over me and tried to help me take a rolled sausage from the tray she held in invitation. I was embarrassed that I had been singled out in such a way but a word from a lady who I had just met stopped the maid's over-reaction, and I managed to cope well with future offerings.

The only person that I knew well was Canon Coalier and he was the only person whom I did not speak with during the cocktails. Everyone else made a point of coming over and introducing themselves. I had seen all these people, but had been somewhat frightened of them before. Now in this house, with the laughter and friendliness, they smiled. A smile can do so much.

Dinner was a sit-down affair. The dining room had two walls of windows that looked out on the Raymonds' large back garden. The shrubbery was beautifully groomed. The leaves swept over the grass with the gentle evening breeze and the last light. The ten of us who remained for the meal sat around a magnificent table set in silver and china and crystal. The maids put down their trays of hors d'oeuvres and served the courses – the shrimps and soup and a wonderful main dish with chicken and rice. The meal itself seemed so easy to eat; the pieces were bite size and I did not have to struggle cutting, or rather tearing, my way through the meal as I often did. The bartender became wine stewart and refilled the glasses with a delicious white wine that sparkled in the ten glasses.

Everything was grand and my spasm seemed very quiet. There was no tension and the conversation ran through many directions. Canon Coalier was a bit out of sorts as his reappointment had not been announced by the church but that seemed the only dark spot that the evening would allow. Someone wanted very much to discuss the assignment by the church to have Pierre Berton write what became *The Comfortable Pew.* His infamous sex article in *Maclean's* was mentioned, and everyone seemed interested in the way Mr. Berton would handle this new topic. I was invited into the conversation but not forced. Most of the time I sat and listened while I looked through the wine glasses and out of the window. My mind wandered but finally returned when I heard my name mentioned, and my future discussed. Mrs. Raymond mentioned what a fine job I had done with the dress I had made her. The three other ladies concurred. The men started talking business. Mr. Raymond, his eyes smiling more than his mouth, led the conversation to things such as equipment and facilities. I sat and listened to these men and women, just some hours and Sunday mornings away from complete strangers, discuss my future in a way that I found not at all degrading as had been the case with institutions.

Someone suggested one of the Sunday school rooms in the basement of the church.

They aren't used all week. I'm sure the wardens would be only too willing to allow Susanne one room for her work during the week.

Mr. Nelson volunteered to look into ways to get me a sewing machine. Customers would be no problem, the church was full of women who were looking for a good dressmaker. Certainly, came the refrain, a chorus of optimism.

Dessert was served. Fresh strawberries and cream and steaming coffee. I had a half a cup of coffee twice and sat quite full and very pleased as the dinner was ended and the serviettes, still creased and starched, were folded on top of the table and the chairs were moved back with sincere compliments to Mrs. Raymond.

Liqueurs were served in the dining room but I refrained. The night had been heady enough already. Mr. Nelson and Mr. Raymond arranged what they thought would be their last golf game of the year. The ladies planned an afternoon of bridge for the following week. The other gentlemen talked about the problems within the church with Canon Coalier. I sat and listened and was happy.

The big grandfather clock in the hall rang its hourly chant. Someone looked at his watch and the party started to break up. How could I thank Mrs. Raymond enough, or all these people? They had done so much more than just give me dinner and help me with my future. So much more, and yet nothing could be said for I didn't know the words. Coats were put on, and hands shook, thank yous conveyed and more compliments offered.

I thanked Mrs. Raymond and her husband and left the door on the kindly arm of Mr. Nelson, who somehow sensed what I felt. It was a dark night, clouds had covered the city during the party. The street lights cut through the black. As they moved around the circular drive the headlamps from four cars shone on the Raymonds who were standing at the door waving goodbye.

I was tired and I melted back into the Cadillac's seat. Mr. Nelson arranged to meet me in two days time when he would have some reports about the things discussed that evening. He seemed so businesslike and yet so helpful at the same time. I was sure that something would be worked out. I watched the trees in the wind and the streetlights until we turned onto Yonge Street. The car stopped at the Y and Mr. Nelson helped me up the stairs.

Goodnight, Susanne. I'll see you in a couple of days.

Thank you, Mr. Nelson.

I waved down to his wife who called goodnight to me from the curbed car.

Thank you very much.

I made my way slowly and awkwardly up to my room. It was so sparse and the furniture was so cheap but it was home and I went to sleep very quickly that night.

Five weeks later the city prepared for winter. The clouds had turned grayer, more threatening, and the rain seemed colder and thicker. People were putting the linings in their raincoats and were wearing gloves. I had my room in the basement of the church and it was perfect for my uses. I had a long table that was ideal for pattern-cutting. The fluorescent lighting surrounded me with a more than adequate if somewhat cold light. I had a new sewing machine that the provincial Department of Welfare had paid for, thanks to the kind efforts of the gentlemen who had attended the Raymond's dinner party.

I had gone to my room in the basement every day for two weeks and waited for orders. I waited for the pay-phone in the hallway to ring and for one of the many women in the church who were looking for a dressmaker to phone and make an appointment. There was some work, but very little. I had made some aprons for Mrs. Nelson but the other ladies had not called. Mrs. Raymond and her husband were on an extended world cruise.

It was November. Perhaps it was a bad time to be starting.

I worked on a new winter dress I was making for myself. The sewing machine was perfect, it had all the latest features and many switches, but on this day I had trouble keeping my mind on what I was doing.

I heard the rain pouring down a drain pipe that crawled down the church. It dumped cold rain beside the small window at the top of the basement room. Even on sunny days, the only light was fluorescent, but with the rain and the silence from the rest of the church the place seemed extra gloomy that day. The telephone hadn't rung in two days. I had eaten my brown-paper-bagged lunch by myself and had read a paperback book.

I was trying to cut a pattern on the long table that the children used on Sunday mornings. There were only a few marks on the table and I had already found them and knew to avoid them while I was tracing patterns. Yes, the room was really ideal indeed for my work. But on this day I had trouble with the scissors, my hands were very shaky and my cutting was poor. I wished that I had been given a key to the church kitchen so that I could make myself some coffee, but I hadn't and the janitor was off that afternoon. I pulled my thermos out of my satchel and with effort unscrewed the top and poured myself some coffee. It was cold and bitter and I put it down and ignored it.

I was so happy to have such a wonderful sewing machine. Mr. Nelson and Mrs. Raymond and Canon Coalier had hounded the provincial Department of Welfare until they sent the cheque over to Canon Coalier. It was a fine machine but I wished I could use it better. I got out the instruction manual and read a part again. The rain seemed to be getting heavier and I hoped that it would stop before it was time to go home.

I thought about the afternoon that Canon Coalier had taken me down to the appliance store on Yonge Street and bought me the machine. We had walked from the Y. It was a glorious day. One had the feeling that it might be the last such day before winter and that it should be grabbed and cherished. I hoped that Mr. Nelson could play golf on such a day, and that Mrs. Raymond's group, if they were playing bridge, would move out onto the patio.

The students were out in their T-shirts and summer dresses and held hands and downtown, where there were no trees, one might have thought it was spring. Canon Coalier was in a happy mood; his reappointment had been announced and he was pleased that both the wardens in the church and the Provincial Department of Welfare had been so helpful in furthering my interests. He didn't seem to mind my slow walking and we talked about many things during the trip and looked in store windows.

We had been advised by the department to go to one certain store where their machines were of the best quality and where delivery would be faster than at some others. It was a big store but soon the Canon had solicited the aid of the manager and explained the situation. The manager himself directed us to the sewing machine section, through the washers and driers, the refrigerators and stoves and the radios and televisions. It looked like a good store, clean with good displays. And the manager was very friendly and interested in what sort of machine I wanted.

Well, Susanne, I have an appointment so I leave you in the hands of this good man. Canon Coalier was gone.

I assumed that he had taken care of the money with the manager when he first met him, when I had stood to one side and looked at the televisions.

The manager's expression changed. He waved over a salesman, said he was busy and left.

I had to explain the situation to the clerk. He decided to check with the manager so he ran off into the back of the store after him and left me feeling altogether uncomfortable and out of place. I stayed with the sewing machines and waited and watched the people walk by the window. Some of them looked in. I saw secretaries and young executives check their appearances in the mirror-like big picture window.

The clerk returned. Very well, these are our machines.

I finally found one that was very good and just a little under the amount of money that the department had given for the machine. But the salesman was not very helpful. I asked him about various features that the display card touted but he was disinterested and said that the manual would explain it all.

I decided on that machine anyway. I was sure I would be able to figure it out myself. The clerk was trying to sell a television to a young couple who were asking a lot of questions that he seemed more able to answer.

I'll take this one, I said.

Yes, just one moment, he said.

I had waited while he continued with the young couple. They seemed unconvinced and walked out. He returned to me.

This way, please. He led me to the counter. He took my name and address and then as an afterthought asked what was wrong with me.

What crippling ailment do you have? He laughed as he said it, but it was a mean laugh.

Cerebral palsy. Would you please have the machine delivered to St. Radegund's Church and not the Y.?

Oh, you don't like to talk about it. What's that address?

I told him. He marked it on another piece of paper and not the bill of sale.

I wanted to leave the store. I had my machine and was glad but I wanted to get out into the sunshine, out into the streets even though some of the people stared at my spastic walk. I signed the bill of sale, and asked him again that it be delivered to the church.

I'm going to be working there, I said.

Yes. I have a note made of it.

The young couple came back into the store and returned to the television section. Another salesman came up to the couple and my clerk rushed away. He didn't say goodbye or thank you.

I had left the store.

The machine had been delivered to my address at the Y, and the manual still seemed incomprehensible. I had been held up and unable to complete a dress for Mrs. Raymond before she left on her holiday.

That had been the last nice day before the cold of autumn. The suburbs were getting frost every night. Outside it still rained and the weatherman had said it could turn to snow before the evening.

I tried to get back to my pattern cutting but still I was unable. It was four-thirty. I usually left about then. If the telephone hadn't rung by now it wouldn't, I said, half to myself, half out loud.

I heard someone in the kitchen and hoped that I would be able to have a cup of coffee before the dripping wet of the bus stop.

I put my materials away and covered the sewing machine. I would work on the manual again that night; I put it into my satchel and gathered my books and my thermos cup and my instant coffee.

The telephone rang.

I opened the door and spilled the cold coffee that was still in the cup. I hurried as fast I could to where the phone was. I turned the corner to the hallway and one of the members of the ladies guild had picked it up. I heard her say hello and listen and then say: I don't know what you mean. Then she hung up.

She looked at me and walked away.

Was that for me? I asked. I was excited and my voice squeaked. She turned and looked at me with blank eyes and then turned away.

She shrugged and walked down to the kitchen. I heard her laugh and then ask whoever she was with why the wardens would let that retarded woman use a room in the church.

Perhaps the phone call hadn't been for me.

I returned to my room and cleaned up the spilt coffee with

some paper towelling. I turned off the light and with great effort locked the door with the rusty key. I was feeling very bad. I pulled myself up the bannister of the wooden stairs to the side door to face the rain mixing with half snow and dusk. I was very cold and damp and as I waited at the bus stop the rain became the year's first snow. Winter had arrived.

A year passed. Winter had turned to spring; it was warmer at the bus stops. It was hot and humid in the summer and the autumn came. The cars had rolled by the bus stops splashing slush and flooded waters to the sewers. They had risen the choking dust of the summer and smashed the dead leaves of fall. Twelve months had passed and my room was still perfect for my work and I had mastered all the features of my sewing machine.

It was November again, another rainy day. The drain pipe had fallen down last spring and had not been fixed and the rain poured from the hole in the eavestrough and crashed beside the window at the top of my basement room. There had been more work but not as much as I had once hoped. It seemed that there were not that many women in the church who were looking for a dressmaker. I still did not have a key to the basement kitchen, and I had been asked to make myself as scarce as possible when there were lunches or gatherings. The telephone did not say hello very often either.

I was becoming a better dressmaker and had gained some steady clients. With my pension, I could make ends meet and had finally moved from the Y. My friends from there still phoned and many of them ordered clothes, but I missed the people at the Y and the fact that I had never had to spend a lonely evening there. Now I did.

I was living in a small, comfortable apartment in a new high-rise development complex. I had wanted something closer to the church but had had difficulty finding such a place. When I decided to move, a placement agency had given me a list of places, small furnished flats in houses. Some of the landlords and ladies had refused to even allow me to see the rooms. There was no point.

Oh, you're handicapped. We don't rent to handicapped people. They closed the door.

Other places were on second or third or fourth floors and the stairs were worn; often there were no stair railings or bannisters and it would have been just too difficult for me to manage the treacherous steps.

I finally found an apartment. The building had a wall of elevators and the rent was reasonable. But there had been so many problems.

There had always been many problems.

Would the rain every stop? I had stayed longer in the church that day. My work was done and I waited for the rain to stop before leaving. The weatherman had promised clearing skies by mid-afternoon. Still it rained.

The janitor was setting up tables for a dinner that evening in the main basement room. I could hear him crashing tables and sliding chairs over the waxed linoleum floor. Soon some of the women would be arriving and I would have to sneak away from their cold hostile stares, escape like an animal from loaded guns.

I wanted to leave the church room that afternoon and forever. Most of the people there were not like those who had gone to the Raymonds' dinner party – how long ago had that been? The church basement was a cold place with antiseptic green walls and faded woodwork, with locked doors and echoing footsteps and muted voices on the other sides of doors. And it had a room where I kept my sewing machine and cut my patterns and waited for infrequent telephone calls. Perhaps in the New Year I would move everything to my apartment and work from there. But that would be more difficult for my customers. And I would have to face the problems of buying a big table and other things.

When I had moved, I found that there were many things needed, that my possessions were meager and not at all sufficient to equip an apartment. I had saved money, and friends had advised that I open an account at one of the big department stores to facilitate my shopping.

I finally found the credit bureau in the store. It was tucked away in hiding, and the women lined up behind cages and waited for their visitors. I stood in line with others, not all of whom were applying for a charge account. Perhaps I was in the wrong place? I asked the man behind me if this was where one opened charge accounts.

I hope so, he said. That's what I'm trying to do.

He was a young man but going bald, well dressed with a wonderful smile. He started to tell me that he had been told to go to three different places and that this was number three. If this wasn't right, he'd open an account across the street.

Yes, demanded the woman from behind the cage. Her hair looked starched and taped like a wig. She didn't smile from behind her smudged horn-rimmed glasses.

I'd like to open an account, a charge account.

But you're crippled.

Yes, I have cerebral palsy.

We don't give credit to cripples, she declared and looked past me to the man with the balding head.

But why, I've got the money?

I began to fumble for the clasp of my purse. I had my bank book inside – proof enough, I thought, of my ability.

Move aside, she demanded.

I stayed where I was and the man behind me did not move either. I looked to him for support but he looked away and moved to the other line.

I found my bank book and shook it out of the plastic covering in front of her. You can phone my bank manager.

We don't give credit to cripples. Her voice sounded mechanical. I stepped aside and leaned on the chipped enamelled counter. I turned my head. People were staring at me, others looked at the ceiling.

Crazy woman, I heard someone say. I put the bank book, its lines neatly printed with my savings through two years to total a thousand dollars, in my purse. I struggled closing its broken clasp and walked back into the merchandise of the store.

Everyone seemed to be staring at me. The elevator was crowded and the elevator operator called me dear when I reached the ground floor.

Oh, be careful, dear, Watch your step, dear.

I said thank you.

I hurried to the street, out the revolving door that always frightens me because people always insist on making them go faster than I care to go, can go. It spilled me into the hurrying lunch-hour pedestrians and the outrage and embarrassment of reflection. I looked at the window and saw myself where the sunlight hit the window. My hands shook, my head shook, my body shook. Someone bumped into me and I almost fell over. He was a big man in a hurry and he just kept going. I leaned against the window, my back against a display of expensive evening dresses and tears came to my eyes.

Tears had often come to my eyes that year.

The rain was letting up, it no longer crashed beside the window, but fell in trickles into the muddy ground. The janitor was still moving furniture as someone, a woman, was giving orders with a high demanding voice somewhere out beyond my closed door.

It was time to go home, to take the bus and subway and another bus, to be pushed and hurried in the crowd and to prepare dinner and watch television and hope that tomorrow would be a better day – maybe the telephone would ring and say hello.

I sat in the window seat of the Gray Coach bus, three rows back from the front. Ahcad of me was the black-haired head of the driver, and farther ahead, unseen, Toronto. I was going back, back to my comfortable but lonely apartment and the next day to the forgotten room in the basement of St. Radegund's. Behind me a crying child, its mother sticking a comforter in its teething mouth; behind me a simple and warm goodbye from my old university friend, Rozanne, a Christmas of joy and warmth in the friendly atmosphere of her parents' home, slow walks in the snow-crusted small town, congenial dinners and remembering and talking in a red easy chair in front of a flickering fire, while outside beyond the frost-covered windows, winter howled its presence.

The bus rattled its way slowly through another snowstorm; some impatient travellers dared the hard-packed passing lane of the 401. I imagined other hectic holidays, the hurrying home to a job and housework, children showing off their new gifts. An occasional station wagon carried a shiny new aluminum tobaggan; I could see down through sedan rear windows children playing with some new game, mothers watching over the seat, interrupting and explaining rules.

It was the end of a year, the beginning of another was but days off. I wished I could have stayed at Rozanne's longer, to share another holiday but there were customers waiting and I had said I would be back. I would have liked to have stayed away but I couldn't. I turned my head back to the storm outside the windows, to the sleepy Ontario countryside, snow covered, naked trees bending only slightly to the snow-filled winds. I watched the dim outlines of the distant farmhouses and barns, dark against the whiteness of the scene, blurred by a frosted window. It was growing darker; I reached up for the reading light switch and after several attempts flicked the cold button. I turned and saw that the baby behind me had fallen asleep, secure in its mother's arms. The bus was quiet, the roar of the motor filled the compartment; there was a rattle in the left rear, occasional laughter from some whispered conversation somewhere behind me.

Laughter. Yes I had laughed with Rozanne during my visit. We had shared laughter.

It was dark out. The farmhouses couldn't be seen; there was an occasional light far away in the countryside. A light from a kitchen window. And inside, a family like Rozanne's gathering around an old oak table, bowls of vegetables and gravy-covered meat. A father saying the blessing, a thanks to God for all there was to be thankful for. A dozen conversations, not one leading anywhere, perhaps not even important to anyone else but those sitting at the table. A mother asking what her children did that day. Children asking if they could watch a program on television after their regular bedtime.

In the seat across the aisle a man snored. I moved over to the aisle seat because the light seemed to be better and Rozanne had given me a book to read during the trip. I leaned and could see up the aisle and out the large front window. The storm seemed more severe through the headlights and we were moving very slowly. A snow-covered sign, its white letters melting to the crusted snow seemed to say Toronto but I could not tell for sure and I couldn't see the mileage number after the name. I heard the driver turn and speak to the couple in the seat behind him.

It's going to be a long trip. I don't know what time we'll get to Bay street. Maybe we won't. He chuckled but it was muffled over the distance to where I sat.

I reached under my coat to find the package that Rozanne had given me at the bus terminal when I left. She had said that I would find it very interesting but would say no more. I hadn't asked any more. If Rozanne said I would find it interesting I probably would. We were still that close despite the years since we had seen each other regularly.

I hadn't wanted to talk about going back, leaving the laughter of their home for the loneliness of my apartment. There had been so few times when I had been content the way I had been that week. I had enjoyed helping in the kitchen, doing the simpler things that I could do. At home I had to do everything and it was rather frustrating.

She had just handed me the parcel and told me it was a book that I would find interesting. I had put it under my arm with a thank you and gone on talking about what I had to do at home and why I couldn't stay. I tried to tell her that I wanted to get back, that I wanted to return to Toronto but I don't think I fooled her. She knew that my tears were more than goodbye tears. Even more than thank-you tears. I had pulled back the sliding window of the Gray Coach and waved goodbye as the bus pulled away from Rozanne.

Keep in touch, let me know how things are going. She yelled above the roar of the first gear. Write me and let me know what you think of the book.

Yes, the book. My hands were cold and I had trouble tearing off the brown wrapping paper. I seemed to be making a lot of noise and was afraid that I would wake up the man across from me but he only moaned and moved closer to the cold window. He looked content through what light there was in the crawling bus.

The book. The book was *Karen* and Karen's picture was on the cover, a girl perhaps ten years old, blond and smiling and pretty with blue eyes. Karen had cerebral palsy and this was a book about Karen written by her mother, Marie Killilea. Rozanne was certainly right in thinking that I would find it interesting.

The storm did not cease. The winds still attacked the bus but I did not notice any longer. I read about Karen and the affliction that we shared, the compassionate approach of her mother, her disappointments and fears concerning Karen's mental capabilities, the progress of a growing mind inside a body that could not respond to a physical timetable, that did not walk when it was supposed to. I read about doctors who had no explanations, the ignorance of family and friends who made their own conclusions. And a mother who would not give up hope, who would not stop with many disappointments and who finally found an answer and was working to tell others of her find.

Karen and I shared so much. I cried in that slow snow storm and relived parts of my childhood – the hunger and eagerness that could not be expressed or if expressed was ignored.

I did not finish the book that night. Soon the brightness of Toronto filled the darkened bus. The man across the aisle woke and lit a cigarette. The monotonous drone of the motor turned through gears on Toronto's snow-covered streets. I placed the book aside and moved back to the window seat. I watched the rows of apartments and small houses turn to stores as the bus travelled the deserted downtown streets and finally stopped in the covered depot on Bay street.

It was two o'clock in the morning. Would my friend William have waited this long for me? I hoped so. I couldn't afford a taxi and the bus lines and subways would have stopped for the night. I wanted to talk to someone about the book. About Karen.

William was waiting for me. He stood in the cold terminal, sleepy eyed, a cup of coffee in his gloved hand. He waved and stood and waited as the bus emptied its tired travellers and finally me. He helped me down the black, plastic-covered steps, went in and got my suitcase and helped me to his car and then through the same streets, all the same, to my apartment.

I told him about the book, but he was hardly able to share my excitement, tired from a days' work, another's looming just hours away. I repeated again that I could have taken a taxi but, no, he wouldn't hear of that. I was wide awake, excited that finally I had read something about cerebral palsy other than the cold, not-so-sure words of medical books. He helped me up to my apartment, almost fell asleep in the elevator, and kindly refused my offer of a cup of coffee.

I was alone. But I wasn't lonely. There was something with me. The apartment had been left untidy by the preparations of my departure. I wanted to do something, to let this thing grow within me. I had to be tired but I was so stimulated, too excited to even consider preparing for bed. I cleaned up my bedroom and unpacked my suitcase. In my study I reshelved some books that were lying on the desk. I pulled out my dog-eared copy of *Black Like Me* and sat down and started reading some of the passages that had always struck me in a certain, almost inspiring way. I pulled myself out of the chair and found *Karen.*

I thought about *Karen,* a book about a child with cerebral palsy, written around a happy family setting. A family like Rozanne's, a child who had not yet reached a stage where she must cope outside of that setting. Could I use my own experiences and report, as John Howard Griffen had, a situation that is not happy? I pulled myself out of the chair again. I was growing tired. My muscles twitched uncontrollably as I walked through my small living room. I paused before certain objects that I had had since my childhood. A china figure that had been in my parents' home, a home not like Karen's. Mine had not been filled with hope and love.

I looked out the high-rise window. The storm had stopped, the city would awaken to a white covering. The snowploughs, with their blue flashing lights, were starting to clean away tomorrow's traffic problems. Men and boys would have to shovel walks so that people could manoeuvre safely through the sidewalks. There would have to be a lot of clearing away. It would be difficult.

I had left my room in the church, left it and the empty halls and the table that the children used on Sundays. I had moved all my sewing materials and equipment to my apartment. I went out very little. Spring had arrived and in the mornings I looked out my window down to the grass and the budding trees and saw a new hope. The pink blossoms in the park across the road grew each day and the nakedness of winter was being clothed in the green of a new season. All the snow was gone from the past winter.

It was over a year since I had first read *Karen* and had decided to try to write about the situation of the handicapped. My condition was not improving, but I had found some refuge in my apartment. Indeed, the sunlight that poured through the windows of my rooms might have been enough to brighten me.

It might have been, but it was not. I could not hide myself away from the world and its ignorant stares, nor would I retreat from my intent to obtain some means of independence that was not based on my pension and the lesser rates that I charged to my friends because they could not afford to pay me what I would receive had I not been handicapped. I suppose that I was being used in some way or another, but I would not begrudge my friends my inexpensive services. I needed the work that they gave me and they had not balked at my move to the apartment. I had given up on the wealthier members of St. Radegund's and did not even like going to the church on Sundays. I still heard the whispers as I descended the stairs alone.

I woke each morning to the insistent buzzing of my alarm. I padded to the bedroom window and drew back the curtains to meet each day – the sunshine or drizzle, the gray clouds or the enchantment of soft white snow flakes as seen from a high-rise window. It was all part of a life that I did not necessarily like but had had to accept. It would be better if I made it better. It hurt and was confusing but it could be better.

I was not alone and I was beginning to see that. I could look down from my window to the park and knew that there were many other handicapped people who shared this imprisonment within bodies that would not function properly. And they too saw the spring spread across the trees and the greening ground and the drying ditches. They wondered why they were not given a chance to use the brain that lay dormant within a body that could not meet certain demands.

I walked past the full length mirror on my way to the bathroom. My hair was messed from sleep and I didn't walk very well because all my limbs shook. My knees were turned into one another and I held my hands in a rigid and claw-like way in front of my body; my head was turned to one side, my neck crooked. That is how the world saw me; that is as far as it could see me. And many like me. We have cerebral palsy, or are crippled in some other way, but we see the buds in spring and it gives us a new hope too.

And sometimes I wonder why.

But I didn't that morning. It would be a full day. I had fallen asleep the night before over an article I was trying to write about the legal status of the handicapped and had not gone to bed until about two. I had a dress to finish that was to be ready for that evening. I wanted to return to my writing.

I soft boiled my eggs and toasted my toast and read the paper. The front-page weather report predicted a high of sixty degrees and I thought that if I had time I would like to go down to the park and sit on a green bench and read and listen to the sounds of playing children. I read the news of the growing American involvement in Vietnam and about the rising cost of living and put the paper aside.

I didn't like my kitchen because it did not get the morning sun and because it always took too long to prepare my solitary meals. I fixed some coffee. My spasm was bad and I spilled some over the side of the cup and on my dressing gown.

I bathed and dressed and went into my sewing room. The dress was almost finished and I was sure that my customer would be pleased. I opened the curtains and turned on the radio to a music station. The hum of the sewing machine's motor mixed with the music and the sunlight and I lost myself in my morning's work. The sun spread through the room and brightened the red of the dress and the blue of the walls. By noon the dress was finished.

I was so glad that I had moved my sewing operation to the apartment.

I made a peanut-butter sandwich and put it in wax paper and went down to the park to eat lunch with the birds that were coming home for the summer. I walked slowly along the cinder track and smelt the freshness of spring. There were some younger children in new spring jackets and black glossy rubber boots. They walked past me and stared as their mothers hurried them along. It was colder than it had looked from the window of my apartment; spring does that – it promises more than it usually delivers. I ate my sandwich quickly and went back to the apartment; the elevator speedily returned me to my retreat above the ground.

I entered my sewing room. The sun had passed over the building and was now warming the apartments across the hall. I took the cover off my typewriter and pulled some material from my cardboard filing box. I sat down in the chair that faced the window with no horizon. Big fluffy spring clouds passed by my sight; they brought me pictures and images – men's angry faces, lambs running and jumping, a white pussy cat asleep in a corner. They passed against a deep blue sky while I sat and waited to go to the typewriter and watch my fingers move to the spasm of my body and the anger in my mind.

I tried to write every day but it was difficult. It would take me a long time to be able to cope with the hurt that accompanied the relating of my experiences. And there seemed very little point. Perhaps it was better, I sometimes thought, to sit and look out the window and allow my mind the fantasy of clouds on a spring day. What I had written and sent away was returned by all the publishers that I had contacted. The brown manilla envelopes and the editors form notes were not encouraging.

My friends had been encouraging but they seemed embarrassed by the content of the articles. That was reasonable. They could not know what it was like walking down a street or riding in a bus. They could never understand how or why the doors had been slammed in my face when I had looked for a job, how each pane of glass and slab of wood had blasted through my memory, or how the chips of glass and wood splinters sat cradled in some cavity of my mind where they rubbed with each day's movement. They hurt me and always would.

I pulled myself out of the chair and sat at the typewriter. I had received it for one-tenth its price from the IBM company. It was custom-made so that I could rest my hands on its slanted keyboard without engaging a key. It was much better than my slow and untidy handwriting and had eased the pressures of trying to find someone who had the time to type my articles for me.

I turned on the light on the desk. I looked at my watch; it was two-thirty. I could write for three hours if I could get started. What had my friend David told me? I must be more objective. I turned the machine on. The motor hummed as the black belt moved around the wheels. I turned it off and the hum sank into the quiet of the room.

There was so much to be said. I was finding more material every time I went to one of the informal lectures that I had been attending at the university. But how could I be objective when I knew that I was a member of a fourth-class citizenry? That I was a member of a group of people who were segregated and ignored. People did not have to give me credit. They did not have to sell me food or rent me accommodation. The handicapped are not mentioned in the Bill of Rights or in the United Nations Declaration of Human Rights.

I had tried to accept this information objectively, to see the consequences of such a state, but I could not overcome the hopeless feeling that it generated. I looked at the world. I saw racial injustice, sickening discrimination for the Black, the Maltese, the Indians, but they at least had their ghettos, their reservations, and an emerging pride. They had something somewhere where they could be respected human beings. And I had nothing. The handicapped had nothing; one cannot call decrepit rehabilitation centres and pity something. Even animals were afforded sanctuary and shelter from cruelty. There was a growing concern for their environment and their battle against extinction.

Where was I? Where were the many thousands of people, handicapped through fate? We came second to the black man, poor and hungry in his ghetto, second to the buffalo, ragged and mangy on his protected range. It was all so clear, so unavoidable: we were but fourth-class citizens in the world community.

I sat and stared at the recessed black keys of the typewriter. Perhaps in time I would be able to push them in the right order, to form the right words, so that I would be able to suppress this rage and force my shaking hands to write something that would make some dint in the crusted shell that surrounded the situation and enclosed the ignorance of a society that could not see where it had never been shown to look.

But shadows were starting to form around my sewing machine and my pattern table and the chair in the corner that looked out the window to the approaching dusk. Where had the afternoon gone? I had wasted it with spring clouds and blank-page rage. It was like many afternoons.

The buzzer in the hallway sounded. Somebody was calling up from the entrance to the building. I hurried to the intercom and pressed the button, straining because it was too high to reach comfortably and I was tense and anxious.

It was my customer. She had been a friend when I lived at the Y and liked to drink tea. I went into the kitchen and put the kettle on. The sun shone through the thin curtains from the west. I looked out the window and down to the flow of traffic, the people going home from their work. The next morning they would be going to work as the sun rose high in the sky from the east. Tomorrow I would try to work again. I went to greet my friend at the door.

Two years later I was on the verge of a nervous breakdown. The pages had for the most part remained blank while the situation had become clearer and yet more shady, clouded with a foggy amount of knowledge that frightened me and increased my inabilities and frustrations to a point where I could no longer cope.

I would hear rumours and stories from people who said they had witnessed the filth and squalor of the Home for the Retarded

Children in Orillia. I had heard about children being whipped, about people with cerebral palsy who were locked away and treated as retarded. I heard about the unhygenic housing facilities that the handicapped were forced to live in, about how their pensions were funnelled right to the directors of the establishments and for the most part withheld from the recipients except for a meagre allowance. Some of this hearsay seemed unbelievable but when I integrated it with some of the things that I had personally discovered it became horribly possible. When I discovered that one of the heads of a Toronto charity for the handicapped did not even know what cerebral palsy was, I became more afraid that even the most grotesque things I heard could be true.

I would return to my apartment and sit and imagine the horror of the situation and grow fearful of my own safety. I would hear noises in the hall, footsteps that seemed to stop at my door. I always kept a light on in the living room and I had another lock put on the door.

I was frightened and I knew that other handicapped people must be frightened. I wanted to express my ideas but it was very difficult. When I did send articles to a publisher they were returned. I didn't eat well and I began losing weight. The only time things were better was when I slept – if I could get through a night without a nightmare – my Uncle Edward coming to get me, my parents behind him with blank expressions, my mother waving a knife.

When I walked down a street I imagined people stopping, becoming inanimate and staring at me. My spasm became worse than I could ever remember it and I was frightened to answer the telephone.

I broke under the strain. It was a Sunday morning and I was in church. I attacked the guest speaker on the sunny steps. He had given a polite sermon when I was expecting something that would attack the complacency that I saw everywhere.

I was expelled from St. Radegund's.

I was referred to a specialist by my doctor who was concerned about my condition.

I had been charmed by my first meeting with my new doctor, his boyish good looks and cute broken English.

Is that what Valium does to you? he asked.

I had never heard of the drug, never in my long associations with other doctors and institutions for the handicapped. He explained.

It's your spasm that makes you build up those tensions. On top of not having the quality of voice to defend yourself against people in the right manner, you also can't express yourself quickly enough. You get all tied up with fears, hold everything back. It's a good thing to blow up, but in your case you store up so much that you could get yourself into jail.

His explanation had made so much sense, and he went to such pains to assure me of the benefits of the drug, that I promised to at least try it.

Just hours after my first experience with valium, I had picked, almost numbly it seemed, a dime from my change purse. I didn't realize that I had even done it until I had handed it to the lady behind the counter at a restaurant. Valium worked. That afternoon I ate a corn beef sandwich on a kaiser, manoeuvring my salad fork with the other hand at the same time. Yes, it worked. I could now manage with relative ease mechanical moves that had seemed either impossible or at least terribly difficult. I had returned for my next appointment with another kind of hope.

He prescribed less sleep, citing my usual nine and half hours as just another reason for the degree of my spasm. I was like anybody in this regard – my muscles were made more flexible by an increased amount of activity. He suggested six hours sleep a night.

I had been progressing well. The keys of my typewriter had been dusted and I was starting to write again. Valium was a miracle.

The drug was expensive – too expensive for me. But I had discovered that I could receive financial assistance for its purchase through the Toronto Welfare Department.

It was time to re-enter the world, to leave my apartment and face the bus stops and the pushing crowds. I had been given the address of the central branch of the Toronto Welfare Department.

The voice from the telephone had told me to go there.

It was a hot day and the dust rose from the streets in choking clouds. The bus was crowded and smelled of perspiring people and oil and gas and I had to stand clutching the warm metal bar and teetering in the packed aisle.

The houses and stores along the route became dirtier and smaller. I got off the bus. I hurried before the doors closed on my slow movement down the steps. I walked between children in tattered clothes throwing stones at passing cars. I walked to the address I had been given.

I entered a large hall – it could not be described as a room. It was poorly lit, with an accompanying dirty floor, a few rows of rough wooden benches and a cast of characters the like of which I had never seen. The women were dirty, slovenly; the men sat on the floor, some with a wine bottle in a paper bag nestled between their legs. I almost turned around and walked out but my own need for money to pay for my Valium somehow overcame the fear.

I was directed to a wicket, given a number, and told to wait.

But there were no seats. I leaned against the dirty wall, as far away from anyone as I could be. I watched the unshaven men as they emerged from one of the doors leading off the hall, their leering smiles as they held up a cheque. They would disappear, only to return to their comrades and share the liquor the government had just purchased. I could not escape the scene, was forced to play when some of the men would approach me with their bottle and offer me a "quick snort." One seemed very intent to force his hospitality on me and only because of the warning of another, much bigger, was I spared such indecency; it was a kind gesture but it resulted only in several rounds of raucous laughter at my expense.

I waited for almost two hours. My drugs played second to liquor. Then, finally, I was shown into a little office. Paint was chipped away at every corner, the floor perhaps dirtier than the halls had been; cigarette butts were sprinkled like party decorations.

I explained my situation to the woman who listened with little interest. I showed her a letter that I had received from the director's office and a note from my doctor. She replied with a rather rude demand that I fill out the appropriate information form, which was very inappropriate.

I waited some more and finally re-entered her dark little office to be told that the department would spend no more than twenty dollars a month for any drugs. I told her that I would be purchasing the drug at a drugstore very close to where I lived and that I really had no idea of what price this store charged for Valium.

She disappeared to find an answer. I sat and kicked cigarette butts. A long half hour later she returned and quoted the druggist's price of $22.50 for a hundred 10-milligram pills. In a calculated tone, which I assume was meant to make me grateful she said that the department would make out a cheque for that amout to the drugstore I had indicated this month and that my case would be re-evaluated for future months.

I proceeded to the drugstore to make the purchase.

I had my Valium when I returned to my apartment but I was angry and humiliated. I unlocked the door. The apartment was hot and I had a headache. Would I have to do this every month, I wondered.

I spent that evening working on a dress but the anger was growing. I was uneasy and tense. I tried to read but my mind would not stay within the pages.

I woke early the next morning. The rain had finally come in the night; it soaked and cooled the city.

At nine o'clock I phoned City Hall. I asked to speak to the mayor but he wasn't in.

The secretary asked if there was any message.

I told her about the conditions at the Welfare Office. I let my anger tremble through the telephone wires.

She said that she would pass along my protest.

I never received a reply from the mayor but the next day I did receive a call from a woman at City Hall. My case had been reviewed. In the future the department would send me a monthly cheque to cover the cost of my drugs and I was free to make the purchase wherever I wished.

(This proved very successful in that I discovered an unexplainable difference in the cost of the drug. It ranged from fourteen to thirty dollars for the same amount. Even at the cheapest price I could not afford an increased maximum dosage, but I decided that it was worth this small extra expense if I would escape similar monthly scenes.)

Two weeks passed. I was recovering my health very well. I was receiving more orders for dresses and the weather had been magnificent. I was watching the six o'clock news.

There was a film story about the welfare facilities at the address that I had visited. Rows of red vinyled seats had replaced the benches; there was a new coat of paint on the rough walls and the camera focused very clearly on the male and female guards who had been posted in the building.

Well, how about that, I said to the television.

Of course, I can never know if I had had anything to do with such a transformation. But I imagined that I did. I needed to see the results of standing up and saying that something was wrong.

I could see the sunshine before I reached the top of the stairs that led from the subway. It bounced off the dirty yellow enamel panelling and danced on the smooth metal railing in front of my pulling hand. Students rushed by me on the other side of the double staircase, others made their way around my slow ascendence. A girl smiled and said good morning to me.

It was November, 1967.

I counted the steps from the subway platform; I hurried so as not to hold up the people behind me. I counted to thirty-seven and wondered about the coming hour. Dr. Rainford had sounded so sincere and interested over the telephone.

Can you come and see me tomorrow at the college?

It had been a long time since I had been to any college. The evening sessions on campus that had once been so enjoyable were years away.

Yes, tomorrow is fine. I'd like to come to the college.

The appointment had been made for eleven o'clock in the morning.

It was a chilly and fresh day with northerly breezes that promised to be winds by the afternoon. I wore a heavy coat that I had made a few years before. It was becoming somewhat worn-looking and old and I decided that I would make myself a new one for the coming winter. That at least would give me something to do.

I struggled through the sticking exit turnstile and headed to the large glass doors that dumped me into the street. It was warmer than when I had left home and I undid the top button of my coat and started to walk to the college.

The new flag, the red maple leaf, hung limp in front of a building across the road. I walked to the corner and stood in a crowd and waited for the light to turn and heard a young man whistling a song that the radio had played all summer – a lively tune that said: we love you Canada.

I had continued my routine of working on dresses in the mornings and writing and reading in the afternoons and at night that summer I had watched the country celebrate its one hundredth birthday. In black and white, on my seventeen-inch screen, I had watched the fireworks, rockets of white light heading for the heavens, slowing and dropping and then exploding and dripping to earth.

I had stayed in my apartment and had written about how the nation neglected its handicapped citizens. But still the publishers were not concerned or not interested, and all the manilla envelopes had been returned.

The light turned green and I waited till the shovers in the crowd had pushed ahead of me and then I walked slowly across the street. The light turned yellow and I had to hurry to the curb, to the safety of the sidewalk. I stopped and leaned against a street lamp pole to catch my breath.

Dr. Rainford had sounded so encouraging. I had to remind myself of his words. I needed encouragement so badly. And I needed it soon.

That autumn had wasted itself away. I had stopped reading and writing and my sewing was becoming boring. I slept more than was good for my spasm. I had stopped doing my speech exercises and would leave the apartment only when it was necessary. Often I let the telephone ring until it stopped.

I had felt my anger turn itself into the bitter daydreams of what could never be. I started to wonder what my life would have been had I been born healthy. I had even begun watching the afternoon soap operas and escaping into the blankness of apathy. It wasn't that I knew what was happening. I had seen nothing, felt nothing. My disappointments were slowly smothering me and I was becoming bitter to the celebrations and laughter that existed outside my lonely apartment.

And then, the afternoon before, I had watched Dr. Rainford on a television program that had investigated the extent of racial prejudice in Canada. I had been very moved and impressed with his honest and sincere manner; he mentioned many of the things that John Howard Griffen had written in his book, *Black Like Me.*

That evening I had phoned Dr. Rainford and received his invitation.

I started to walk toward the campus. It was twenty minutes to eleven.

The sidewalk was not wide enough for the many rushing students. They spilled into the street and blocked the honking cars. Boys ran and pushed and dodged between pretty girls who hugged books to their chests; they tripped over narrow curbs and laughed down the street.

I had to walk slowly and carefully. I measured every step. One young man, his head intent in a large book, ran into my rigid arm. He stopped, looked up, looked at me and then returned to his book and walked away.

It was a slow walk but fortunately it was not a long way to the main building. I stood on the huge cement patio in front of the raised front doors and waited for the between-class rush to stop or at least let up before I grabbed the railing and started up the narrow stone steps.

I waited in the sun and watched tomorrow's leaders and wondered if they would do things differently or if they would do different things.

Could I help you ma'am?

The voice came from behind me. It was slow and hesitant and deep.

I didn't need any help. I could make my way up the steps and open the huge glass doors. I was all right.

I turned around.

The boy smiled at me.

He was a big young man, almost fat, and he wore a dirty plaid jacket and faded jeans with a rip in the knee. His hair was long and greasy and he had pimples on his forehead and for a second I thought he was ugly. And then I saw the smile.

I didn't say anything.

He looked concerned.

I'm sorry. I thought maybe I could help you.

I explained. I have an appointment with Dr. Rainford. I'm to meet him in his office in ten minutes.

I know where his office is. Could I show you to it?

Thank you. That would be very kind.

He crooked his arm and I took it. I folded my rigid spastic arm around the boy's strong plaid arm and walked up the stairs. He went slowly and deliberately. He introduced himself as Ernie and told me that he had a class with Dr. Rainford and asked if I'd seen the professor on television the day before.

After he had held the doors and escorted me into the building, Ernie took me to the elevators and explained that he would have to find a janitor. Students didn't get elevator keys, he said with a laugh, but it was worth the trouble because Dr. Rainford's office was on the fourth floor.

I waited where Ernie left me until a man came at me jingling a ring of keys.

Why can't you use the stairs like everybody else, lady?

I didn't say anything. I would have used the stairs, of course – if Ernie hadn't offered to help, if Ernie hadn't gone to so much trouble.

Would you open the door please, said Ernie.

The man snarled and mumbled something but fulfilled the request.

We walked into the elevator and the door slid away the sneering face of the janitor.

Ernie apologized.

I could hear the quiet mechanism of the elevator; it mixed with my new friend's shuffling feet and the hollow din from outside the capsule. Then, for an instant, movement stopped. The doors opened to a pale yellow wall and a worn, blue carpet and a hall that was empty. We escaped the elevator. Students sat outside doors and chatted along the corridor.

It's this way, directed Ernie.

He took me to Dr. Rainford's office and knocked softly on the door.

Come in, sounded a voice.

Ernie opened the door. There's a lady here to see you, sir.

The door opened wider and Dr. Rainford appeared.

Miss Moss. I'm so glad you could come. Do come in.

He took my hand very gently into his palm. I knew that I was glad I had come. His face was one that a television camera could not capture – the harsh lights could not hold the gentle Creole features and the laughing, tender eyes.

Please come in, Miss Moss, he repeated.

I turned to thank Ernie before I entered the small office. I glanced to the left and could not see him. I then turned to the right, to see his large back and his slow ambling stride as he moved noiselessly down the corridor.

Thank you, Ernie, I called.

He turned and waved and smiled and walked backwards for a few steps and then disappeared around a corner.

There are some good people, Miss Moss.

I turned to Dr. Rainford. He smiled with a tenderness that choked my response.

I moved to the chair that he held for me and collapsed after my exhausting walk.

Dr. Rainford started to ask me about the articles I had been writing, what the subjects were about. I had brought one of my last efforts for his inspection and I sat and stared out the window behind his black wavy hair as he read my short article. I watched a shadow move across the opposite building and tried to see something in the expression of the man who sat at the desk across from me.

Finally he put down the last page. He removed his glasses and leaned back in his chair and brushed his hand over his face.

I didn't say anything. I waited until his eyes had come down from the ceiling.

He started slowly, measured each word.

I think, maybe, we need to take this out of Canada and put it in the hands of an American publisher. I think I understand why none of the publishers that you've contacted have chosen to print your material.

Is there something wrong with it?

No, not really. Nothing that couldn't be fixed. It's just that it's a little hot for a publisher up here who hasn't had experience with this sort of thing.

I'm going to see Griffen in January. Maybe he can suggest something.

Griffen? Dr. Rainford asked.

Oh, I'm sorry, Doctor. John Howard Griffen, author of *Black Like Me.* You mentioned the book on television yesterday.

Yes, of course, but how are, why are you seeing him?

A friend of mine knows him quite well and he's arranged a meeting when he comes here to speak in January. Doctor Rainford nodded.

You must be excited about that. Yes maybe he can help. It certainly won't hurt to try. But don't worry, even if he can't help, we'll get something going. It's the kind of problem that needs attention. Shall we have some lunch?

Dr. Rainford took me to the cafeteria and over lunch we talked about many things – my early life, my attempts to secure a job both at home and in Toronto. His eyes seemed to suffer with me and I thought that perhaps we had shared some similar wrongs.

Your story should be told, he said.

The cafeteria was very crowded and we sat at a little table in the middle of the large room. I struggled with a tasteless hot dog and felt the stares of many spectators. But it didn't matter as much as it usually did. I drank coffee from a styrofoam cup that twisted as I forced it to my mouth. And yet inside I felt a strange and welcome calm.

Perhaps we could get you a place on a television show, he suggested. *Take Thirty,* or no, even better, *Pierre Berton.* I think he might do it, I'll start to look into the possibilities of that.

I wasn't sure. Television? Me, on television?

Yes, you Susanne.

I didn't pursue the subject. It overwhelmed and frightened me and I didn't want to talk about it. He noticed my fear and suggested we wait until after I had met Griffen.

It was almost one o'clock. Dr. Rainford looked at his watch. I'm sorry but I have a lecture this afternoon and I must meet a student at one-fifteen. I'll walk you to the front of the building.

We walked through the halls in silence as we dodged the running students. I looked at Dr. Rainford once and smiled. When we reached the front of the building, he held the door for me.

I'll let you know what's happening as soon as I hear anything. And please, phone me at any time. Here's my home phone number.

He gave me a number with his name clearly printed on the torn off corner of a piece of blue-lined yellow paper.

Anytime, he repeated.

I walked out the door and turned and said thank you.

I turned from his smiling tender eyes and carefully walked down the stone steps.

The sun was at its highest in the deep blue sky of the fall afternoon. The wind had increased and the flag at the front of the building whipped and buckled and the girls' hair flew from their grinning faces. I walked back to the subway, back towards home and the typewriter that awaited me.

I smiled and I remembered many of the things that Dr. Rainford had said. And as I walked I looked at all the young men to see if one of them was Ernie.

Dr. Rainford had been so right. There were some good people.

I couldn't wait to get home, back to my apartment and an unfinished article that had been shoved away and almost forgotten in the crowded top drawer of my desk.

December 11, 1968.

The alarm sounded at seven A.M. It crashed through my restless sleep, insisted that I wake to the dreary day. It was dark in my bedroom. Slowly I reached for the cord of my bedside light. I pulled it unsteadily and the light glared into my sleepy eyes. I closed them in sudden pain.

My stomach was restless, butterflies woke with the alarm. They attacked. I pushed myself out from under the warm covers and made my way to the bathroom. I was nervous. Perhaps I could keep busy most of the day. There was a great deal to do. I wondered how many people would come that evening. Perhaps the show would be taken off at the last moment.

I went back to the bed. It looked so inviting. The quilt that I had made was rumpled and the indentation in the pillow called to me. I went over to the window and opened the curtains. It was still dark outside and down below the street lights still shone in the brisk morning air. The traffic had started. I had eleven hours to wait. I walked through the rest of the apartment and turned on lights; shadows raced from the 60 watt bulbs. Out the study window the sky started to brighten but it was only the growing of grayness.

I turned back to the room and slowly walked to the coffee table where the weekly television listings lay disarranged and slightly crumpled. I sat on the springy sofa and picked up the sheets of newsprint. My eyes raced through the blurred listings, they sped down the columns and finally seized on six o'clock, channel eleven. There it was: *The Pierre Berton Show* with Susanne Moss.

I pushed myself off the couch, walked into the kitchen, and put the kettle on.

Would it really happen, I wondered, as I sat shaking at the kitchen table. The clock on the stove said seven-twenty. It would be a long day. I tried to read the paper. Nixon was starting to say things about Vietnam. Still the bombs were falling and the men dying. I turned again to the television listings for reassurance. I was reassured.

The kettle had boiled, steam crept up the kitchen wall, it moistened the pink paint. I got up and unplugged the black cord and made my instant coffee, my half cup. I tried to read Richard Needham but I couldn't. The hollowness in my stomach would not fill with the steaming coffee. I stared at the paper, page seven. I would have to go out at some point in the day and get some cheese and crackers, and there were a few things that I needed for the dinner I would serve.

I wondered about the reaction to the program, about what it would mean to my future, and about the future of the handicapped citizen. How much could I do? I had been trying to do something for three years. I had sat and struggled with the words and only increased the material that I kept in my filing box. I sat at the table and stared out the window, at the endless horizon of morning clouds, the grey turning to an even and dirty white. I would be glad when the day was over, when the year was over and another would start.

I was thirty-three years old and wrinkles were starting to line my face. Perhaps it was time that I accomplished something; perhaps this program would be the start and 1969 would be a new beginning.

Perhaps.

It had been a depressing year in many ways and yet it had been the most encouraging year of my life as well. I had met John Howard Griffen.

How many times had I read *Black Like Me,* travelled with the author through the south of his homeland, his skin washed to blackness, his mind becoming even more troubled about the peculiar nature of black-white prejudice? He had come to Toronto, sickened by the effects of the drugs he used in his experiment and yet healthier than most people would ever be in a more important sense – he had stood up and said what had to be said, had been the subject of hate because of his work and had remained brave and proud.

I cannot put in words my feelings on that night. I met Mr. Griffen and sat with him before he gave his address. When our hands touched at our first meeting it was as if something very good and almost holy was transmitted from his weakened fingers. I had trouble talking; I was choked by the emotion of the moment. I listened to him address the huge gathering that had crowded into the hall. He stood throughout his lengthy talk, his cancerous bones never yielding to a more comfortable position, his steel-enforced jaw never ceasing to the pain he must have endured.

He spoke about his past, what he had seen as a white man turned Negro, how he had felt neither a black man nor a white-educated writer, but something in between that he himself had created by changing the pigmentation of his skin. He spoke about the repercussions, the threats that he and his family had endured since he made his honest report. His voice was grave; it was a grim story.

I listened and I let inspiration form my thoughts. If this man could be brave, could stand up and say what must be said, why couldn't I? Why couldn't I discount my petty financial troubles and stand up to any imagined retorts? I was afraid to hurt those I loved, those who had helped – they were my only concern.

The sad voice of John Howard Griffen had changed to one of hope. It has been worth it, he said; worth it because he was greeted by crowded halls and heard by thousands who were acting.

I made my decision. I vowed that defeat would only make me try harder, that someday I would say what had to be said about another social problem.

Mr. Griffen had had to leave immediately after his address, but we did have time for a short goodbye and my very understated thanks for what he had personally done for me that night. I gave him three of my articles with the hope that he find the time to read them and comment – after having met the man I wanted his advice more than ever.

I had received a letter from him in two days. He had spent the time on his flight out of Toronto with my work and his reply. He suggested that the best way for me to proceed was to write a book. He said that I needed help and was sorry that he himself was so committed at the time; he would like to assist me in such a project.

I had received a great deal of assistance from Dr. Rainford. With his encouragement and assistance I had started this book. Valium was still doing wonders and I felt able to accomplish almost any physical task – that was, of course, not the truth but it almost seemed to be.

But my spasm was bad on the morning of December 11th. I watched my hand as it reached for the coffee cup. It shook convulsively, with no control. I grabbed the cup with two hands and pulled it to my mouth. The coffee was cold. I got up and dumped it into the sink and plugged the kettle in again. I walked into the study and turned on the radio. It was almost eight o'clock and time for the news. I still listened to CFRB but Jack Dennett had replaced Jim Hunter.

1968 had been a bad year in the news. I had listened to America, its assassinations and riots – Martin Luther King and Robert Kennedy, both senselessly slain. There had been days when it was all so depressing. But the news passed away after the funerals and eulogies and the world continued. The black man remained repressed, Vietnam felt the pounding of bombs, protest remained disregarded.

I turned the radio off in the middle of the sports reports. I did not want to listen to the news that morning. I returned to the kitchen and made another half cup of coffee. It was eight o'clock; I had ten hours to fill.

I had started the book in July. I had wrestled with the memories of my childhood, with the sheets of carbon paper, with the slow pounding of the wrong keys on my typewriter.

And I had quit in July. I had watched the riots in Chicago, the swinging billy clubs of white-helmeted policemen, the blood of the children, and the tears of the reporters. What was the sense of saying anything?

And the following Sunday, in warm blue-skied Toronto I had been accosted by a policeman on my way to church.

I had been approaching the subway, dressed in a new summer dress when a policeman had stopped me.

What were you drinking, lady?

I was humiliated by his very public accusation and indignant that this kind of thing would happen to me while on my way to church in Toronto. (I had been stopped once before by the police but I was bundled for an outdoor excursion in the middle of winter and the policeman had been most apologetic when he learned I had cerebral palsy.)

People streamed to and from the subway station. As I stood to one side, this huge policeman bullied his way into my life on this fine summer morning. How could he have overlooked the pretty new dress that I had just finished making the night before? How could the prayer book and the hymnal have escaped his attention? I know that some people may think that my manner of walking is the stumbling of a drunkard or a drug addict: I can see the stares everywhere I go. They haunt me and frighten me, for I can never know what lies behind them. Some, no doubt, are curious stares, others show pity; there is finally this last kind, so real and terrible on that ugly morning – the embarrassing accusation that my appearance is something I have inflicted on myself.

What were you drinking, lady?

A few of the morning subway crowd had stopped to watch. One disreputable-looking character, his face unshaven, his knees rubbery, had gawked from behind the policeman's left shoulder. I stood alone. I wanted to run, but I can't even do that. I went into my purse; the Valium seemed not be working, my hand shook violently. I pulled out a crumpled letter from my doctor that I carried just in case anything like this might happen. The policeman read the letter.

Sure lady. Cerebral palsy. He grinned to his audience.

Okay, you can go, he said. He flipped the letter back at me.

But I hadn't gone to church. I turned and walked back to the apartment. Tears had mixed with the sunlight and blinded me. At home the sunlight had sprayed through the study. The beginning pages of the book, hours of work lay on the table. I had picked them up and crumpled them, torn them with my shaking hands.

What was the use?

I finished my coffee. I had started the book again in August. Dr. Rainford had shown me that I could not quit.

It has to be said, Susanne. Because it is, it has to be said.

I walked into the study. There were now almost a hundred pages of the first draught. There was a dress on the long table, almost finished, just a few little things to do. Perhaps I would have time that afternoon. No, I'll have to vacuum and dust and that is a half day's job. And I'll have to cook and prepare cheese and crackers. Go out and shop.

It was eight-thirty. I went into the bedroom and got ready for the day.

I grew more anxious throughout the day. I had faced the cold dampness of December, waited for the buses and made my purchases. I had pulled out my old vacuum cleaner and slowly walked it through my small apartment. I had dusted the furniture, prepared a meal, and set the table for a buffet dinner. And it was only four-thirty. And I sat and waited for the first guest.

William and his wife Mara would be the first to arrive. He had said he would come right from work. It would be better with people in the apartment. Jill and Larry would be there about five o'clock.

I looked at my dress and decided to change into the one I had worn for the taping. I walked into my bedroom and changed but my hands were shaking so much that I had trouble finding the small zipper handle and pulling it up the side of my dress.

It was silly to be so nervous. I hadn't been nervous during the actual taping of the show. And it had taken so many months to arrange my appearance. Dr. Rainford had helped so much. And Mr. Berton had been kind and friendly.

We had sat at the familiar table behind the homey coffee mugs and the cameras had blinked their red lights while the director sat behind the large lighting stands. It had all gone so quickly and then it was done. And then the wait had started until this day – December 11th.

I finished dressing. The alarm clock beside the bed said quarter to five. I walked back to the living room and into the kitchen;

everything seemed to be ready. Mara would help me with some little things that I was unable to do. She could cut the cheese and William would serve the sherry.

I sat down and flipped through my dog-eared copy of *Karen.* It wouldn't be long, I tried to tell myself, but each minute passed too slowly. I got up and looked down at the moving traffic, at the lines of cars on the street below me. The street lights came on. The buzzer rang. I hurried to the intercom. It was William and Mara. I waited outside the door, waited for their warm smiles. The elevators were so slow. They finally came from around the corner in the hall. William was whistling and smiling. He carried a bottle of sherry.

Are you nervous?

Yes. I laughed.

They came in and we talked in the kitchen while Mara arranged the cheese and crackers. The others started to arrive – friends who through many years and tears had helped. Everyone was excited. The time passed quickly with nervous laughter. I played at being hostess but I kept looking at the clock on the kitchen stove. What if the program were cancelled at the last moment.

I asked Larry.

Don't worry, Susanne.

But I worried.

Someone turned on the television. It was ten to six. Come on Susanne. I put it off. I checked the dinner that sat in the oven. It looked all right but I wondered how it could be.

Susanne, we've got you a seat here.

I went into the living room.

Here sit beside me.

I sat down. William took my hand. A program was just ending. The credits were given, rolled across my small black-and-white television screen with happy music. The room was quiet. No one was saying anything.

We waited through a detergent commercial. I tightened my hold on William's hand. I clutched it through a cigarette commercial.

The music rolled with a shot of a skyscraper. The lettering came across the screen; *The Pierre Berton Show.*

The familiar voice of Bernard Cowan announced:

This edition comes to you from Toronto.

The camera switched to the studio, to the long table, the back of Berton's head. Susanne Moss, said Pierre Berton. The camera turned on me.

My grip relaxed. I would finally say something. Finally people would be listening.

Part III

Part III

The telephone rang just seconds after the program ended. It would not stop ringing for the next several days. Of course, many of the calls were from people I knew, but the vast majority were placed by others, interested people who had seen the show and were impressed that someone of Mr. Berton's stature had finally interviewed a handicapped person, and that I had spoken honestly of what the handicapped person is forced to endure.

The first calls I received that evening were from people whose trembling was evident through the receiver. They were moved by the show. Many mothers asked that I speak to their children while many of these children, a few as young as seven-years-old did not even attempt to hide their tears. I would finally be forced to change my telephone number to an unlisted one, but this evening I enjoyed speaking to these people. The fact that they called was a kind of success. I only hoped that something more significant would be achieved.

The anxiety that had been so obvious before the program was gone. I only had time for a few mouthfuls of dinner between the merry rings of the telephone. People were reluctant to go home. Others started to arrive. There was a second airing that evening after the late news and my apartment was even more crowded for it.

Dr. Rainford arrived and he watched the program in disbelief.

Susanne, you finally did it. That was all he could say. Tears choked his words.

The last guests left about one o'clock. I was alone. Cigarette butts filled the ashtrays. Glasses sat empty on the tables. I had wanted to clean up myself and had refused the offers of help. I wanted to think about the evening, to remember each moment – the laughter that had sounded in my small apartment, the many phone calls, and the congratulations.

I cleaned up. I did it slowly. I was in no hurry. I must be tired I thought; it had been a long day but I didn't feel tired. I was too excited. A calm had come over me. I seemed almost relaxed. I went through the apartment and turned off the lights and sat in the dark living room while the lights from the city shone peacefully through the windows.

It had been a very satisfying night. I liked the recognition, the congratulations, and the phone calls of gratitude. But with the faint light was the gnawing doubt that nothing had really been accomplished. It could never be enough if the program brought me recognition, while what I had to say was ignored. That was not the goal, never the objective. I hadn't spoken just for me, just for my personal goals and frustrations. I spoke for all the handicapped. They deserved much more than my recognition.

I went to bed. I wrapped the covers around me, buried my head in the pillows and waited for sleep.

Would the handicapped receive anything? I prayed that they would. And I fell asleep.

I was awakened the next morning by the telephone. It would interrupt all my activities for the next several days. Many people phoned, young and old, people in all manner of occupations, ministers and clergy from all denominations. They all expressed their appreciation for what I had done. I was stopped on the street, addressed in stores, my mail box could not hold the letters that the postman delivered each morning. Everywhere was appreciation.

But I did not want appreciation, I wanted action. I hoped for understanding, public information. I wanted jobs for the handicapped, the demolition of segregated housing projects, and the abolition of demeaning workshop employment. And I received polite thank yous.

I knew that my appearance on the *Pierre Berton Show* could only be a first step but I had hoped for more encouraging results. It didn't take long for even the recognition to end; it seemed that appreciation was all that would result. That soon ended as well.

Perhaps my initial doubts as to the accomplishments of my appearance on television were only indicative of the mood that challenged me all through 1968. My mind swung like the pendulum of an old clock, regimented to the mechanics of the world. There seemed to be no escape.

Yet I was wrong to discount any good. True, segregated housing did not cease, the workshops did not close. But as that year finally departed with the raging storm of New Year's Eve and as I applied myself to the job of studying and answering all the letters that I had received since the program, I realized that in some small way something had been accomplished.

Mr. Berton also received a great many letters about the program. Most of them were short notes of appreciation, thanking him for being the first talk show host to interview a handicapped person. About a quarter of the people who wrote agreed with my statement that there was just no available means for people to gain information about the handicapped; it seemed to be one subject that had been categorized as too controversial, out of the mainstream of the many troubles that our society was forced to handle. (Indeed, one woman wrote rather ruefully that she had heard of cerebral palsy but that she had always assumed that it was some kind of new household gadget that was beyond her budget.)

Many of the letters addressed to both Mr. Berton and myself encouraged the writing of this book; it appeared that many people wanted more insight into the problems of the handicapped. They were interested in what I said; they would like to hear more.

This was very encouraging; it was a new incentive. I returned to the long job of placing my life story on paper with the determination that such encouragement from the public can create.

The program's success brought subsequent discussion with Mr. Berton and his encouragement to get on with my book. I found this a rewarding recompense, but more important this continuing dialogue enabled me to discuss a point that he had voiced during the program. The handicapped person, especially one who has muscular difficulties, is the leper of the new age. We are regarded as loathsome creatures, who have in some way sinned and who live each day with the curse of our affliction. The ignorance of such an attitude has not been overcome since the biblical age and this only increases the frustration that the handicapped person must, indeed, is forced to live with.

Everyone familiar with the stories of the Bible will know the connection between leprosy and the palsy and the devil's curse. It is perhaps unbelievable – I find it maddening ignorance – that such a connection might still exist, only revised to the times. The handicapped lives his life as one cursed by this same tailed and horned creature, a repulsive and loathsome individual. It is the outlook of an Uncle Edward; one that breeds on all that is repulsive in the intellect of man. One can go on forever citing the absurd elements of such an outlook, but one can never deny that it exists. It does.

And the handicapped live each day knowing that it does.

The letters that I received bore strong proof of this fact. And so many other facts, shameful and sickening. I read each of the letters that I received, answered as many as I could. I read many letters from people with muscular difficulties who asked about Valium. (I had made a great point about my wonder drug on the program.) I could not believe the ignorance of the people who had sent these letters, the seemingly incompetent treatment that they received from their doctors, if indeed they had doctors. I remembered the many visits that I had made for consultation when I was a small child, and the lack of answers. I was twenty-seven years old before I found out the name of my affliction. I wondered if that was not still the problem of many of these people who wrote asking about the drug I used and yet seemed not even to know the name of their affliction. I read pitiful lines in scrawling, often illegible handwriting:

My arms move when I don't want them to.

And there were the militants, handicapped people who wrote and expressed protests as strong or in many cases much stronger than mine. There was no hint of apathy in the strongly worded letters, yet I wondered why these people, extremely able in the art of communicating, had not made their protests more audible. What had happened to these minds that they were forced to protest only to one who had publicly expressed the same opinions? The handicapped needed such people and yet I suspected that they were all cowed into a state that made open protest an impossible and frightening thing.

Very few letters from the handicapped were encouraging. In the main they were filled with ignorance or hollow rhetoric. But they appreciated my words; I hoped that their determination would grow with time.

Parents of handicapped children wrote. One couple wrote that they were considering aborting the child they were expecting because they were both cerebral palsy victims and they feared for their child, the life that they knew awaited the product of their love. (In fact, as I wrote these people, there was every reason to expect that their child would be wholly normal as the possibility of having a handicapped child is the same for any couple. But I wondered if this was really their concern or did they know this fact and yet envision how their child would have to grow up with parents who would never be accepted.)

Letters from parents in western Canada seemed to suggest that the attitude toward the handicapped was even more barbaric in that part of the country. People wrote and informed me about beatings administered by education authorities in attempts to keep the handicapped children away from public schools. And finally, as a last word on the problems that parents faced, one mother wrote me and explained how at times she wished she had given birth to a coloured child, or even a dog. At least then her cerebral palsied offspring would have some guaranteed rights.

The letters angered me, they made me cry. They still sit in a cardboard box, pitiful reminders of individual worlds that I do not know, troubled minds that seek escape from the injustices of our society. No, I do not know them. I have but an expression, sometimes sad, other times unbelievable, of one minute in these lives. There are letters in that box that made me blush for their embarrassing and tasteless content. (One woman wrote to ask me if I had a menstrual period, as if I was some freak who, on top of being considered a loathsome creature, was not even a woman.)

One letter sits on top of the rest. It is from a young man who suffered from the same prejudices and discriminations. He wrote about seeing me on television, about the realization that my words had developed within his own thinking. He had decided to take his life after finishing his letter. He wished me luck and hoped that I would continue my crusade. Perhaps, he said, years or even months ago he would have fought along with me, but now it was too late, the fight was gone with the will to live. He ended the note with one sentence: "I think that not knowing would have been so much better."

He didn't sign his name. There was no way of checking on the authenticity of the letter or the drastic end that the man had intended. I often think about this letter, about the hopeless state that education forces on the handicapped, about the only escape that this man could see. I too had faced the same conclusions but had, through my belief in Christ, determined a different course. I think about it when I hear the brave, complacent words of our national anthem:

"Oh Canada, glorious and free."

And all those people who sing the song, at their football games, at their hockey games. They salute their country – in many ways it deserves their salute – but I'm afraid that far too many of them believe the words.

Probably the greatest immediate benefit that came from my appearance on the *Pierre Berton Show* was the many invitations I received to meet and talk to handicapped persons who lived within the sheltered compounds that I had denounced. This was a relatively new experience for me. My determination to live a normal life and my past history of attending schools with the healthy members of society had kept me from seeing how bad it was. I started this round of engagements with a determination that proved very naive. I wanted to incite these people to protest, make them more aware of their situation and encourage them to start to build a different and better way. Instead I found very little material for protest. It was as if my own words about segregation and the detrimental effects of such a policy were only hollow and superficial warnings beside the real results. Was I too late? Many times I think I was. I am.

They listened to me, polite and listless. When I suggested that they demand the government give preferential hiring to the handicapped, they asked what would happen to those members of society who were whole and unemployed. They didn't seem to want training for more meaningful occupations, but when I asked them why they worked for five dollars a week weaving baskets, they in turn asked: What else is available?

They told me, some of the braver ones, how they were constantly threatened, their jobs and pensions placed in jeopardy by officials and family as means of holding them to their subservient places. They told me, as I noted their rather rude way of addressing everyone by their first name, the repugnant tone, mocking and somehow sad when they referred to themselves and others as either "C.P.s" for those who had cerebral palsy, or "wheeliers" for those restricted to wheel chairs, that they had been taught to act in such a way, to ignore all commonplace dignities, the kind that, if even superficial, lend some sort of respect. But there was no respect; life seemed such a chore to these people. Through the conditioning that they had received, the absurd and childlike environment that they had always been forced to live in, they could see no other life.

I snapped at one of them; I was no Susy the C.P. but Miss Susanne Moss, a woman who had cerebral palsy. He seemed quite stunned that I would not play his demeaning game. Likewise they could not accept the need to seek their own interests, but remained cowed by those who they regarded as more significant, those who were not restricted as they were. Oh God, such visits made me angry.

I met other handicapped people who had jobs, and who to a certain extent contributed as full-fledged members of society. But their involvement was far less than what most people could find tolerable. Yes, they made money, but what good was money when it was so difficult to spend it as they wished? Many told me of experiences like my own – so many years ago in Woodstone – when I had gone to the best dress shop in the city to purchase a gown for my graduation ceremonies but had been refused service in the store. They wanted respect, but could never find it. They were forever reminded of their differences, addressed as "dear," not "madam" or "sir."

For the most part these handicapped men and women realized that people were fundamentally well-meaning in addressing them in such a manner, in grabbing them and escorting them across streets, in pushing them into empty seats on buses and subway cars, but they resented the silent implications that they were not capable of taking care of themselves. They wanted to function as individuals. Everywhere they met only frustration in attempts towards this goal. (One girl told me that people would often come up to her on the street and ask her personal questions pertaining to the symptoms of her handicap. These "well-meaning people" were in fact insulting her. She remarked that "it was as if I asked a fat woman if her girdle was tight.")

None of these people had found any comfort in the real world. They told stories about the cruel way they had been treated in high school and how in most cases the teachers had ignored the situation. I felt very lucky that I had not been subjected to the same thing as it seemed quite commonplace. I talked to one school teacher friend of mine about this matter only to find that it still exists. She told me about a girl at her school who everyone, teachers included, called Limpy.

In my contacts with all handicapped persons I noticed that they were always restricted in their physical abilities by improper medical attention. I couldn't believe how many told me that it was impossible to find a doctor whom they could consult without being accompanied by a member of their family. Most of them shied away from therapy; they had never been informed of the benefits that might result from proper exercise. Everywhere I met this incredible ignorance. Yet hadn't I had enough experiences with doctors and other officials that I should not be shocked by these hopeless stories?

My real research had started. Previously I had read the books, compiled the statistics, visited the projects, but seen only what I was supposed to see. But these were the people, pitiful and angry or listless and ignorant. These were the lepers, the loathesome creatures. They were lonely, miserably lonely, depressed and sullen, often without anyone to share thoughts and hopes, even opinions. (The women are the most lonely; 95 per cent of handicapped women do not marry, while 95 percent of men do. One could postulate several theories for such a situation; mine is simply that women are more compassionate, while men have been raised for the most part to revere a woman's body. It is but one more example of a complex situation; people are swayed by the superficial while overlooking the important. The mind is ignored while the peculiarities of the body serve as the measuring rod of a person's situation.)

Oh, Canada glorious and free, indeed. And for whom?

1969 was filled with one question: why does such a situation exist?

I still do not know the answer. I have tried to find it. I visited the handicapped, sat and talked with them in bare-walled rooms. I heard their stories, felt the depression of their words.

They were not like me. Not really. I could find a new hope in a spring day. I was busy with my sewing jobs, with writing my book. They had nothing. They could see nothing. Their eyes were masked to the green of the spring, blinded by the blankness of an endless winter where flowers never sprang from the rich brown earth.

It was a hot summer. I worked in my apartment and I sweated in the humidity and the sunlight that came into my study. The book progressed through the first draft and into the second. I went wherever I was invited. I hoped to find some contradiction, someone who had risen above the status of fourth-class citizen but I never found that person. Instead I started to read the publications and watch all the television documentaries. I found more examples – but worse.

I read in the newspaper about Marvin Nash and his accomplishments as a leathercraft expert, his goal of starting his own business. Mr. Nash had graduated first in his class from a Toronto technical school, but could never set himself up in his own shop because of the restrictions placed on all handicapped people by the administrators of the handicapped persons pension. I had never known that the pension was cut off if and when a handicapped person had a net income (pension included) of $1,620 and liquid assets of $1,000. This is the policy of the government, a government that professes to encourage private industry and yet restricts Marvin Nash from this same objective. It is impossible for anyone who wishes to start his own business to gain any kind of security with such restrictions. Banks and other lending institutions are unwilling to lend the money to a handicapped person. Marvin Nash was doomed. He could never escape the workshops or the discrimination that existed if he worked for someone else. He could never gain the dignity that he sought. The system would not allow it.

I read about the shooting of Donald Oughton in California. Mr. Oughton was a handicapped person who when stopped by the police and questioned could not communicate because of a speech impediment. He went for his identification and was shot to death by the policeman. The police chief went before the national media and admitted that the policeman had assumed Donald Oughton was going for a gun. But there was no gun, only a dead Donald Oughton, the victim of a dreadful mistake.

And finally, the cruelest demonstration of all, shamelessly presented (or so it seemed) by CBS Television on their program *Sixty Minutes.* It reported a wonderful new German measles vaccine which was being tested in Texas. But they didn't use guinea pigs, or white rats, or chickens. No, they were using retarded children to test the often fatal effects. And no one seemed to care.

But I cared. I cared about Marvin Nash and Donald Oughton, about all the nameless children who were being used as testing devices. And the more I cared, the more I cried. I found more to cry about.

During the year I came into contact with a community college in the Toronto area and became involved in a study that a class of students was conducting into the conditions at institutions for the mentally retarded. I talked to the various students and their teachers, heard them recount tales of children being intimidated by the staff, and beaten. To quiet the tantrums that resulted, the disturbed children were thrown into cold showers. The students told me that some of these children were not retarded at all but had cerebral palsy, or other learning disabilities. They had been buried within these institutions by Uncle Edwards, doomed to an existence that forced them to mental retardation. I tried to persuade these students to make public their findings but met with only an apathy that I could not understand from the young and idealistic. The report was worded in unobtrusive language and forwarded to the government official in charge. The students had done their project, had received their mark. That was enough.

For them, but not for me. I contacted an officer of the Ontario Human Rights Commission. I told the man what I had learned from the students and demanded some satisfaction from my protests. I was outraged. This was 1969, the atomic age, the welfare state. It was supposed to be an age when man had overcome his barbarianism. I remembered the horrifying tales that Uncle Edward had threatened me with, that my parents had on occasion used to keep me subservient to their narrow wishes. They were true, still, years and years later. And they would remain that way unless somebody did something. An officer of the commission told me, very matter of factly, "we do not consider the mentally-ill human beings because there is no mention of them in the United Nations Bill of Rights."

WE DO NOT CONSIDER THE MENTALLY-ILL HUMAN BEINGS.

That polite forum for the big powers, that not so polite circus for the African nations, that magnificient show piece that is so ironically named the United Nations did not consider the mentally-retarded as human beings. And neither did Canada.

I was reminded of an article I had once read in *Chatelaine* magazine by Tori Salter, her inside report of a hospital for the mentally-ill.

Miss Salter was a registered nurse turned writer who had herself purposely interned in such an institution as a temporary depressed patient. She wrote about the lack of dignity afforded the patients, how many had been committed by only the certificate of one doctor but were in fact perfectly well or could be with proper treatment. But there was no proper treatment. The patients were cramped like rousting chickens, overworked as maintenance personnel, punished when they dared to protest such treatment.

Miss Salter followed this article with a more recent example of the abuses of the system. She wrote about Lettice Edwards who had been legally restricted to such an institution for fourteen years, committed by the whim of her aging mother and one doctor. Miss Edwards was perfectly normal and only escaped and made the case known after she had cleverly worded a letter to a lawyer who came to her rescue. The letter had to be so worded because every letter coming out of the institution was inspected by the officials.

In Canada, this same article went on to explain, a person can be committed to a mental institution by any so-called "responsible person" and one or two doctors. Cerebral palsy victims fall easy prey to such a procedure because of the physical similarities between the two afflictions. Even the much-toted review-board procedure proves meaningless, Miss Salter explained, because in many cases the patient is so confused by shock treatments or drugs that he is unable to make a convincing showing before the board of examiners.

Epilogue

Place: A studio of the Canadian Broadcasting Corporation in Ottawa.

Time: January 1, 1970.

Pierre Elliott Trudeau, Prime Minister of Canada, addresses the nation in the customary New Year's Day Address.

Susanne Moss is watching him on television, the flower in his lapel, the round dimpled cheeks. He switches between French and English, is very polished, very political. He smiles and frowns, reads his address.

Miss Moss is falling asleep and the she hears him say, his pronunciation very crisp;

"There is no segment of our population which is condemned to silent, hopeless oppression."

She gets up from the chesterfield and turns the television off. She wants to kick the screen, to drive her spastic leg into his smiling mouth.

Is the government unaware of the plight of the handicapped, the mentally retarded and the confusing indistinguishable mix that society has created?

Is there no hope for the handicapped?

There is so much ignorance of the situation.

Place: A school for the mentally retarded, Toronto.

Time: Anytime – now, yesterday, tomorrow.

A twelve-year-old boy, handicapped in such a way that one

> assumes he is retarded, sits in front of a typewriter. He has never shown any of the teachers, any of the administrators of the school that he is aware of his environment. He never communicates. He has always sat sadly by himself. He is one of the hopeless cases.
>
> A young teacher observes the boy in front of the typewriter, hears his slow beating of the keys. She is afraid his frustration over the mechanics of the machine will upset him, drive him to some sort of tantrum. She approaches, remembers how her textbooks told her how to treat such a situation – be patient, try to explain very simply how the machine works. Bring him back to the other children, to the smearing of the finger paint, the excited laughter.
>
> She comes nearer. He doesn't turn around. She looks down at the carriage of the machine, at the clean white sheet of paper, the almost perfectly typed sentence:
>
> WHY DID GOD MAKE ME LIKE THIS?
>
> A large glistening tear falls from the child's puffy cheek. It falls from his listless world to hers. It blots the word God.

It is a touching story, true and very real. But I cannot blame God, even beseech him. My accusations are directed to men, to those who ignore the situation of the handicapped and to those who condescend and pity.

I obtained a pamphlet from the Canadian Cerebral Palsy Foundation. There was no mention of the intellectual needs of the cerebral palsied individual, there were no stated goals, no emphasis placed on developing the intelligence of these victims or training them for meaningful positions in society. But, there was a great deal of information about the history and funding of the organization, about parent groups. There was finally a plea for public pressure on the government. But for what?

This kind of information will only continue the same policies at a more ambitious level. I have seen what this means. It means that the handicapped will be coddled, segregated to a comfortable environment that restricts, degrades and finally destroys. We don't want this. We want to be citizens of our country, to make a contribution, to live our lives despite our handicaps. We are not incapable. Yet society has imposed such an assumption.

Place: A theatre in New York City. It is the occasion of the Emmy Awards Program.

Time: May 8, 1969.

Jimmy Shulman, a young retarded boy has been nominated for an award for his supporting role in the television play, *Teacher, Teacher,* but the academy has announced that it has disqualified Mr. Shulman from the competition because of his retardation. The benign academy has determined, instead, to present Jimmy with a plaque, a tribute to the young man's fine performance.

Susanne Moss, watching on her small old black and white television set is angry and disappointed by such a pronouncement. She waits for the lesser triumph of Jimmy Shulman. She knows that he will show the millions of viewers that he is a human being, not some despicable animal. The cameras continue to show the young actor in the audience, a handsome, well mannered young man. In one of the shots he holds the plaque – the academy will not even allow him its public acceptance.

Later in the proceedings *Teacher, Teacher* wins an award. A representative of the production unit walks to the platform to accept the small statue. He mumbles a rather unsatisfactory thank you to the presenter; he walks to the rostrum, stares at the cameras. His face shows bitterness and hurt; he projects that to the audience – those in the theatre, those in their homes. He delivers his message with a gripping forcefulness. He tells why Jimmy Shulman was not allowed to compete for his award, how the academy had discriminated against him – barred him from the competition because of his limited mental capacity.

Is it Jimmy Shulman who is retarded? Or is it a world that cannot even see the possibilities of a person like Jimmy making a meaningful contribution?

Jimmy Shulman's tears fall on the world. Society wipes them away without notice.

There are too many tears. They fall from too many eyes and they mask the world to too many people. They cloud and fog the beauty of the earth.

Tomorrow's blue skies are grayed by the humiliation and frustration of yesterday. Today is but a lonely existence. We want to see beauty, to feel self-respect. We want to wake to the hope that it will be. Is it too much to ask? We have paid with too many tears.